Communicating Hope

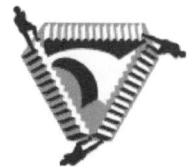

Communicating Hope

An Ethnography of a Children's Mental Health Care Team

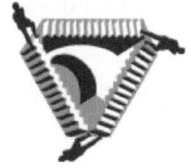

Christine S. Davis

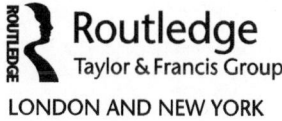

Routledge
Taylor & Francis Group

LONDON AND NEW YORK

First published 2013 by Left Coast Press, Inc.

Published 2016 by Routledge
4 Park Square, Milton Park, Abingdon, Oxon OX14 4RN
605 Third Avenue, New York, NY 10017

First issued in paperback 2017

Routledge is an imprint of the Taylor & Francis Group, an informa business

Library of Congress Cataloging-in-Publication Data:

Davis, Christine S.
Communicating hope : an ethnography of a children's mental health care team / Christine S. Davis.
   pages cm
   Includes bibliographical references and index.
   ISBN 978-1-61132-123-4 (hardback : alk. paper) —
ISBN 978-1-61132-125-8 (institutional eBook) —
ISBN 978-1-61132-708-3 (consumer eBook)
1. Psychiatric social work—Case studies. 2. Mentally ill children—Services
   for—Case studies. 3. Social work with children—Case studies. 4. Child
   mental health services—Case studies. I. Title.
      HV689.D385 2013
      362.2083—dc23
                              2013004765

ISBN 13: 978-0-8153-4653-1 (pbk)
ISBN 13: 978-1-61132-123-4 (hbk)

Contents

Preface   7

Chapter 1: Pizza Party: Defending, Explaining, and Introducing   11
   The Defense   11
   Project Background   12
   Definitions and Explanations   15
   Research Focus, Approach, and Role   17
   Research Methodology   20

Chapter 2: *R. M. S. Titanic*: Meeting Poverty and Disability
Face to Face   23
   Poverty Sucks   24
   The Initial Meeting   27
   Help Him   34
   Another World   35

Chapter 3: Abandon All Hope: Challenging Hopelessnes   47
   Challenging Deficits   47
   The Dollar   50
   Does the Family Have Dreams?   51
   Things Are Going to Get Harder   56

Chapter 4: Appearances Are Deceiving:
Constructing Turning Points   65
   Team Building   65
   Digressions and Crises   66
   Doing What's Best   67
   Boundaries and Limits   70
   Crazy Is as Crazy Does   71
   Express Yourself   73
   The Future Is Now   77
   The Turning Point   80
   I'd Lose It All   86

Chapter 5: Union Gives Strength: Constructing Hope   95
   Undersized and Starved for Affection   95
   Constructing Hope   98
   Continuing to Feel Supported   98
   Collecting Bills   113
   Information Broker   113
   Something to Write About!   118
   Positive Changes   126
   As People with Stories   130

Chapter 6: All Things Are Possible: Hoping and Helping   131
   You're Influencing My Services   131
   There but for the Grace of God, Go I   135
   Emotionally Insecure   136
   Deeper into the Mind-Bending Universe   138
   Those Dominant Hierarchies   149
   They Promised Me Help   150
   Behavioral Control   150
   Trying to Get Home   156

Chapter 7: Team Voice: Constructing Voice   157
   Subtle Doesn't Work   157
   It's Crazy Out There   169
   Feeling More Hopeful   169

Chapter 8: Blended Voices: Constructing a Future with Hope   187
   Transformed   187
   Crossing Boundaries into the Future   189
   Hope, Empowerment, and Support   191
   No Expectations   194
   Voice on the Table   196
   The Moment of Truth   198
   Last Words   209

Chapter 9: Children's Mental Health Practice Considerations   215
   Systems of Care in Children's Mental Health   215
   System-of-Care Principles   215
   Ramifications of Research   217

References   229
Index   237
About the Author   241

Preface

This book is dedicated to the "Stewarts," the "Center for Children and Families," the staff at "Washington High," and the team ("Mr. and Mrs. Stewart," "Kevin," "Alan," "Mr. Camelini," "Jane," "Nancy," and "Peggy"). It is especially dedicated to the memory of "Warren" and all the children, families, and professionals working to raise healthy children in our world today. It is also dedicated to my loving and supportive husband, Jerry, and to the memory of my parents, Arthur and Margaret Salkin. This book is also dedicated to the God of grace, who gives blessings, hope, and help without regard to worthiness or productivity.

Welcome to this story about my experience with a children's mental-health treatment team. This book represents a narrative ethnography of the 16 months when I was involved with this team.

This book has four intended audiences. The first audience is graduate students who want to know what conducting ethnographic research for a dissertation is like. I hope they catch the excitement I felt as I moved through the process of planning, collecting, and analyzing the research. The second audience is health communication scholars who want to learn what interdisciplinary health care teams are like, and the third audience is group communication scholars who want to understand the experience inside an interdisciplinary team. To the last two audiences, this is a story of a bona fide team, and it shows both the messiness and the richness of how a diverse group of people—formal and informal providers from multiple organizations and multiple systems, an adolescent "patient," and family members—came together to work toward a common vision of moving the child and the family forward toward wholeness.

The fourth audience is people in the children's mental health care field—current providers and students studying the children's mental health care field—who want to understand the struggles that families and professionals face. To this audience, especially: please don't read this book as a model for perfection. This book shows you the reality inside one system of care. I have great respect for the team, and the family, but all of us are human. The book is intended to take you into one team, with human beings who struggle with getting it right, viewed through the eyes of one researcher who thought she knew—but had to learn—humility, compassion, and strengths-based vision as she worked through this research. The research is not intended to show you how right we are; it's intended to show how difficult it is to do it right but yet how possible it is to help children and families as we work through the messiness together. Having said that, I hope all audiences will appreciate the grace, compassion, and artfulness displayed by the team (including the family) as they moved forward to construct hope.

Most names of people and organizations in this story have been changed. For the few places in which I used actual names, I received permission from the participants to do that. I have edited and fictionalized specific details and situations for confidentiality and narrative coherence. However, as I did that, I attempted to stay true to the constructed reality of the situations as I experienced them and as they were told to me by my research participants. For my data, I observed team meetings and interactions between team members, conducted multiple interviews with team members, and led three focus groups with the team. I audiorecorded and transcribed the interviews and focus groups and took field notes of my meetings and observations. The conversations depicted in this book came from my observations, field notes, interviews, and focus groups. I "cleaned them up" and edited them to create a narrative, but I endeavored to retain the original meaning throughout.

I attempted to include the voice of all participants through multiple interviews and focus groups, but I understand and acknowledge that my voice as a scholar is privileged in this book. I also understand and acknowledge that I cannot fully understand or convey the standpoint of people with other backgrounds, experiences, and statuses from mine.

This research was done under the supervision of the university IRB, and all participants gave informed consent.

Acknowledgments

This book is based on my doctoral dissertation research and was supported in part by grants from the Center for Mental Health Services in the Federal Substance Abuse and Mental Health Services Administration (#5-HS5-SM52250-05 and #5-HS5-SM52250-06).

I wish to gratefully acknowledge the love and hope given to me by my husband, Jerry, without whose support my dreams would never have been achieved; my mentors, Carolyn Ellis and Buddy Goodall, for their encouragement, confirmation, friendship, and inspiration; my friends and colleagues, Barbara Eudy, Deb Breede, Peggy Davis, and Jan Warren-Findlow, and my daughter, Robin Kumako, and sisters, Kathy and Kelli Salkin, for their support and encouragement. I would also like to thank the faculty at the University of South Florida, especially Ken Cissna, Art Bochner, and Eric Eisenberg, for their incredible mentoring, encouragement, inspiration, and support and my colleagues and friends in the children's mental health field, especially Robert Friedman, John Mayo, Marsha Lane, Norín Dollard, Keren Vergon, and Mary Armstrong, for their encouragement and support. I also recognize and thank my colleagues in the Communication Department at the University of South Florida, the Department of Child and Family Studies at the Louis de la Parte Florida Mental Health Institute, and the Communication Studies Department at the University of North Carolina at Charlotte, as well as my graduate research assistant, Emily Tamilin, for her help in revisions on this manuscript. And, I want to thank God, who makes all things possible: "For surely I know the plans I have for you, says the Lord, plans for your welfare and not for harm, to give you a future with hope" (Jeremiah 29:11).

I hope you enjoy this book. I hope you learn from it. And, I hope it gives you hope!

Christine S. Davis
March 2013

CHAPTER 1

Pizza Party: Defending, Explaining, and Introducing

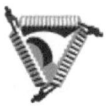

The Defense

I balance five large pizza-shaped boxes as I navigate my way into the Communication office and drop them in the waiting area chair.

"Hey, pizza! For me?" Steve, the office guy, asks.

"No, sorry," I respond, wondering if I should have brought the office staff some food also. "It's cookies. For my committee. I'm defending my research proposal this morning."

"Oh, sweetening them up, huh?" Steve answers with a wink.

"Yeah, you could say that!" I answer. My voice drops to a whisper. "I'm so nervous!" I confess to Steve as I sink into the other empty chair and smooth my jacket. I take several deep breaths and hope the knot in my stomach will go away before they call me in.

"Hi, Cris!" Carolyn opens the door to the conference room and smiles at me. "Ready?"

"Sure!" I say with a confidence I don't feel.

Steve reassures me as he helps me pick up the cookie boxes. "You'll do fine," he whispers.

"What's in the boxes?" Ken, one of my committee members, asks as I carry them in.

"Open them and see," I say as I give a box to each person. Each contains a giant chocolate chip cookie decorated in the college colors of green and gold. Large letters proclaim "Thank You!"—a tribute to the mentoring given to me by the committee members for the past three years. As Eric, Art, and Bob, my other committee members, break off bites of their cookies, I open my folder and pull out my notes.

Carolyn speaks first. "We thought your proposal was very good," she begins. "But we have some questions about the research you're planning to do."

I take a deep breath, pencil poised, ready to write their questions and prepare a response.

"First, Cris," she says with a reassuring smile, "we'd like you to give us some background to this project. Tell us about the research you've been doing that leads to this research you're proposing today."

Project Background

I nod. "For the past three years, I've been conducting research with the Center for Children and Families [Davis, 2008; Davis, Dollard, & Vergon, 2009]. They're a 'system of care' program" [Stroul, Blau, & Sondheimer, 2008; Stroul & Friedman, 1994]. I look around the table. It's a program that offers mental health services to children with SED and their families.

I pause as I look around the table, aware that not all of my team members are steeped in the children's mental health jargon. Ken takes my cue.

"What specifically do you mean when you say 'SED'?" he asks.

I read the definition from my notes. "SED stands for 'severe emotional disturbance.' It's an umbrella term that refers to a mental, emotional, or behavioral disorder that significantly hinders the child from fully functioning in the family, school, or community."

I look up at Ken. "Children are identified as having SED either by the school system or by a psychologist. They've typically been diagnosed with disorders such as Attention Deficit Hyperactivity Disorder [ADHD], depression or other mood disorders, conduct disorders, or anxiety disorders, or a combination of those [Halfon & Newacheck, 1999]. In our research project the children range in age from 4 to 18 years—the average age is 12—and are in the mental health care system because of a history of psychiatric hospitalizations, physical abuse, sexual abuse, running away, suicide attempts, and substance abuse. In addition, their biological family histories include family violence, mental illness, psychiatric hospitalization, criminal convictions, and substance abuse. Children with SED and other mental or behavioral disorders typically have multiple needs and are receiving services from multiple agencies and organizations, across domains such as education, social service, juvenile justice, health, mental health, vocation, recreation, and substance abuse."

"How prevalent is SED?" Ken asks.

"According to Halfon and Newacheck" [1999], I answer, "between 17 percent and 22 percent of children under age 18 have been diagnosed with some form of mental illness, and mental illness has been recognized as a major cause of childhood disability. Almost 7 million children between 9 and 17 years old have SED" [Faenza & Steel, 1999]. I pause. "It's a big problem. Children's mental healthcare costs are the most costly children's health expenses in the United States. Miller and colleagues [2012] refer to the skyrocketing children's mental health costs as a public health crisis. And people with mental illness have less power owing to less political and economic power, fewer policy options and less accessibility to services, diminished rights, lack of knowledge about their rights, an inability to voice their own needs, difficulty in navigating the system, and a lack of knowledge about possible services [Kelly, 2006; Payne, 2009; Stylianos & Kehyayan, 2012]. In fact, some research I was just reading said that access to children's mental health services is so limited that parents put over 12,000 children in the child welfare and juvenile justice systems just to get services" [Child Welfare and Juvenile Justice, 2003]. Ken nods.

"One other thing you need to know is that systems of care in children's mental health are team-based approaches. Systems of care use interagency child and family planning teams in which a team of parents or caregivers, professionals, and informal supports meet regularly to coordinate and plan services for the child and his or her family. Informal supports might include extended family, neighbors, or clergy. Professionals might include therapists, juvenile probation officers, case managers, family advocates, and school representatives. In practice, child and family teams are pretty changeable, with some participants staying in the group the whole time and others joining the group temporarily as needs dictate [Duchnowski et al., 1993; Eber, Nelson, & Miles, 1997; Myaard et al., 2000; VanDenBerg, Bruns, & Burchard, 2003]. Individual child and family team members also regularly interact with the child and family outside of team meetings as they assist and support the family in working through their treatment plan. As some of you know, for the past three years I've been involved in a research evaluation studying the child and family team process through conducting observations of team meetings and interviews with family members."

I glance down at my notes. "We've observed 118 team meetings with 5 different case management agencies, 33 team leaders, and 91 families" [Davis & Dollard, 2004; Davis, Dollard, & Vergon, 2005].

I look back up at the committee. "In the research I've been conducting, I've noticed that these meetings play a strong part in constructing
and reinforcing either positive or negative realities for the family. In the
worst examples of child and family teams I've attended, team members
ignore the family's cries for help, delay services, and criticize and blame
parents in what seems like a power play to define the identity of the child
and family as one of disempowerment, marginalization, and dependency
[Barton, 1996]. In some teams, the team reinforces the traditional power
relations of the medical model of care and in effect renders the child
and family 'muted' [Ardener, 1978; Orbe, 1998; Wall & Gannon-Leary,
1999], making their communication less important than the communication of other people in the meetings."

"Are all team meetings like that?" Bob asks with an exasperated tone
in his voice.

"Fortunately, no," I answer. "When the teams work the way they're
supposed to, they help the family to reconstruct a measure of control in
their lives. When children are diagnosed with a disability, families have to
make sense of the diagnosis and gain control over it, as they adapt to give
their lives order and purpose again [Seligman & Darling, 1997]. Families
of children with disability have to deal with doubt, confusion, and despair
while navigating opposing tensions of joy and sorrow, hope and hopelessness, supervision and control, and love and anger" [Kearney & Griffin,
2001; Sari & Altiparmak, 2012]. At their best, these child and family
teams help them to do this."

"That's great," Bob notes.

"When families have available resources to take care of a stressful situation, they perceive stress as manageable rather than as a crisis. I think
that's one of the key functions of the system of care child and family
team—changing a crisis to a manageable situation by helping the family to
acquire new resources, learn new coping behaviors, reduce the demands
on them, or change the way they view the situation" [Seligman & Darling, 1997].

"How do they do that?" Carolyn asks.

I pause for a second as I think. "When their meetings adhere to the
system of care philosophy they're supposed to follow, they seem to exhibit
what Bogdan and Taylor [1989] call 'the social construction of humanness,' in which people without disabilities value and love people with disabilities as unique human beings. Bogdan and Taylor suggest that treating
people with disabilities with closeness and affection; crediting them with
cognitive ability, intelligence, and understanding; seeing them as unique
individuals with different personalities, preferences, feelings, and life histories; and viewing them as being able to contribute something to the

relationship, helps to maintain the sense of their being fully human. Some researchers have found that helping people with mental illness to be seen as fully human reduces stigma and negative stereotypes [Martinez et al., 2011]. In the best examples of child and family team meetings I've observed, team members do this. Team members know the family members personally and show knowledge of and respect for their unique culture, beliefs, feelings, and preferences. They treat them with respect and even affection. They accept them as equal partners in the team with ideas to contribute. When they're able to take an active role in their own care, that reduces stigma as well" [Stylianos & Kehyayan, 2012].

Definitions and Explanations

"One more question," Ken says. "You mentioned a 'system of care philosophy.' What, specifically, do you mean by that?"

"Well," I say, "to understand what a system of care is, it helps to understand what it isn't. Traditional treatments for mental illnesses are based on many different approaches. A biological approach, for instance, supposes that mental illnesses have genetic, biological, biochemical, or neurological causes, or a mixture of these. This method tends to treat the genetic, neurochemical, and viral factors that are believed to cause mental illness. Biological treatment interventions include psychiatric medications" [Scheid & Horwitz, 1999].

I take a breath and slow down. "An illness viewpoint assumes that psychiatric symptoms, or certain behaviors or behavioral patterns, indicate mental disease. Some people claim that this attitude pathologizes people who don't act in socially appropriate ways and labels them as deviant. In other words, some critics say that using behavioral symptoms to diagnose mental disorders turns what's really a socialization process into a medical issue. Another view, the psychological point of view, regards mental illness as a problem in cognitive and personal factors [Horwitz & Scheid, 1999]. The treatments for this approach tend to focus on helping clients gain insight, relearn mental representations, enhance self-actualization, or improve family dynamics [Peterson, 1999]. These approaches could all be called 'traditional medical models' of care because they emphasize a problem orientation in which people with mental illness are seen as being deficient and responsible for their problems. The medical model stresses cure—a dominant, paternalistic physician role in which it's the physician's job to fix the patients and tell them what's wrong with them—and a passive patient 'sick role' in which the patient is supposed to do what the doctor says to do without questioning [Pettegrew & Logan, 1987; Szasz, 1987; Wampold, Ahn, & Coleman, 2001]. This perspective contributes to a picture of the child and family as being dependent. This model of care typically uses clinical jargon, professionalized diagnostic instruments, and a priority on diagnosis or labeling of the illness" [Barton, 1996; Marks, 1999; Seligman & Darling, 1997].

I smile. "There's a French philosopher named Foucault [1995] who studied power in healthcare and mental illness, and he would say that, in the medical model of care, the patient's body is a target of power in which professionals disempower and marginalize people who are ill and disabled and foster dependency in them."

I glance at Bob. "Now, in the system of care model, that is all turned upside down. The system of care philosophy was developed in the early 1980s in response to several criticisms of the health, social, mental health, and educational systems that said that these systems had an oversimplified, isolated, and fragmented view of crisis prevention and family support [Friedman, 1994; Stroul & Blau, 2008]. Mental health care systems following this approach take a holistic, contextual approach to treating the child within the framework of her or his social, behavioral, and environmental factors. This philosophy encompasses child- and family-focused care, family involvement as full participants in service planning and delivery, family empowerment, individualized care, community-based decision making and service management, a strengths-based approach, and culturally and linguistically responsive care [Dunst & Trivette, 1996; Faenza & Steel, 1999; Lourie, 2008; Stroul & Blau, 2008; Stroul & Friedman, 1994]. As I said before, a collaborative interagency planning team that includes the child and family as full team members often is a part of accomplishing this vision" [Lourie, Katz-Leavy, & Stroul, 1996; VanDenBerg, Bruns, & Burchard , 2003; Walker & Bruns, 2003].

"Cris, why don't you explain to the committee what a strengths perspective is?" Bob asks. "It's a very important part of the system of care philosophy and one striking way that this philosophy differs from the medical model of care."

"Sure!" I respond. "The strengths perspective is a particular departure from the medical model's reliance on deficit language, labeling, and pathologizing. In other words, the strengths perspective doesn't look at what's wrong with the child or family, and it doesn't focus on diagnoses labels" [Laveman, 2000]. I look down at my notes. "I especially like the way Saleebey [1996] puts it. He says that this perspective looks at individuals and families in light of their 'capacities, talents, competencies, possibilities, visions, values, and hopes, however dashed and distorted these may have become through circumstance, oppression, and trauma' " [p. 297].

"But, Cris," Art says, looking at both me and Bob, "you can't just ignore people's problems, can you?"

"That's a great point," I say. "People practicing the system of care philosophy don't ignore problems. They just don't focus on them. I'll quote Saleebey [1996] again. He says that it's 'as wrong to deny the possible as it is to deny the problem' [p. 297]. In the strengths approach, providers use language that moves beyond problems to acknowledge wisdom, abilities, and resources. Providers don't think about an individual's personal identity in terms of deficiency; instead they think of capabilities. They identify existing sources of support in the person's natural environment so that they're looking for what they do have instead of what they don't have [Bronfenbrenner, 1979; Saleebey, 1996]. People using the strengths approach also don't assume that the problems are necessarily rooted in the individual. Problems can be embedded in society, culture, and family [Liegghio, Nelson, & Evans, 2010], and this type of approach often develops interventions that focus on the impact of social conditions and social policies as much as on individual behavior."

I glance at my notes. "So, systems of care operate under a strengths approach in which they acknowledge problems but focus on the wisdom, abilities, and resources that the family has now and what they can—or will—have in the future. Providers don't think about an individual's personal identity in terms of deficiency; instead they think of capabilities."

Research Focus, Approach, and Role

Carolyn asks the next question. "Could you please explain your research question and what you want to find out in this research?"

"In a nutshell," I say, "I'll be studying a child and family team in a children's mental health system of care. I want to understand how the team members deal with shifting from a traditional medical model to a system of care orientation, and I want to understand what the experience feels like for all the team members. I don't think it's possible to comprehend the challenges team members struggle with, just from observing meetings or interviewing a few parents, and I don't think it's possible to study the team's system from looking only at the members individually. I've been looking at snapshots of team processes. I now want to look at one team in depth, longitudinally. To fully grasp how these team members construct reality and meanings for themselves and for the team, I want to research the experience from many eyes, to hear it from many voices, and to see it from many angles, individually, interpersonally, and systemically."

"What's your theoretical approach?" Carolyn asks.

"The approach I'm taking in this research—social constructionism—is a philosophy that says, in a culture, we construct, or build, ideas and meanings about the way things are through communication. That communication can be interpersonal, or it can be mediated through television and other mass media. What we think reality is—and what we think the consequences of that reality are, and should be—is a social construction. It's created through the way we communicate."

Carolyn nods. "What, specifically, will you be looking at?" she asks. "What's your research question?"

"Specifically, I'll look at what reality and meaning a system of care team constructs for the team members and for the team as a whole, and what they do communicatively to accomplish this."

"Tell us more," she encourages.

"I'll look at what the experience is like, from the point of view of all team members and from the point of view of the system, or team, as a whole, to understand their experience philosophically, practically, and emotionally." I take a breath and slow down. "I want my research to help team members to better understand one another. I want people who work in the children's mental health field to better understand the reality from within a system of care team, and I want interagency team members to better understand what it is that they do when they are helpful to the families and what it is that they do when they are not," I add.

Eric sits forward. "Cris, how will this relate to other work on team-based organizing?"

"Although research on team-based organizing suggests many benefits to a team-based approach [see, among others, Cohen & Bailey, 1987; Guzzo & Dickson, 1996; Kayser, 1994; Senge, 1994], this type of approach in systems of care can be quite a challenge. In system of care teams, team members, agencies, and systems have to learn to work together in ways that represent fundamentally different paradigms from their more traditional training and experience [Walker & Bruns, 2003]. I want to understand how the team does that."

Eric leans back in his chair.

"I'm going to study the system of care team in their system or social-world context so that I can fully understand their internal group communication and interaction patterns" [Butterfield & Lewis, 2002; Jacobson, 2003; Sykes, 1990], I say.

"What, exactly, will your role be with this team you're studying?" Ken asks.

"I'm going to attempt to replicate the system of care model in my research. Just as in systems of care they try to give the professionals and families equal voice, I'm going to attempt to equalize the power relation-ship between my research participants and me by making a conscious effort to include the voice and feedback of all of the participants I'm studying" [Hawes, 1994; Reed-Danahay, 2001].

"That sounds great, Cris," Ken responds, "but what will your role on the team be? Will you be participating in team meetings or interactions?"

I pause momentarily as I think of how I want to answer this. I've antici-pated this question and have thought a great deal about this. "I do plan to have a role on the team, but my role will be as a researcher. Just as a thera-pist in her team role has certain behaviors to perform, I as a researcher will have certain behaviors to perform also. As a researcher, I will perform less active, more observational behaviors."

I pause for another minute as I think about what my role has been in these teams in the past. On the one hand, I've conducted dozens of team meeting facilitation training sessions around the local community [Davis, 2005], so most team leaders in these child and family teams have been trained by me. On the other hand, I remember what my boss said when I began doing that training: "How are you going to make sure that your role as trainer won't interfere with your objectivity in observing meet-ings?" Now, as then, I think that objectivity is an illusion and that every researcher comes into the research process with biases, preconceptions, and frames of reference. I think what's important is that the researcher writes reflexively—that is, she includes herself and her thoughts and points of reference [Hertz, 1997] so that the reader understands where his or her bias comes from. Yet, I also think that studying communication in a naturalistic setting requires avoiding interfering with the setting as much as possible.

"So does that mean that you won't participate in team meetings?" Ken clarifies.

"I plan to participate by observing and taking notes," I respond.

"You talked about meetings in which the team was oppositional to the family. What will you do in a meeting if you think the team is treating the child or family badly? Won't you feel the need to say something? How can you ethically sit back and just let it happen?" Ken challenges.

"I've thought a lot about that," I respond. "Sometimes, it's hard to remain quiet. But I think that I can do more good by keeping within my role of researcher and not interrupting the meeting. If I start interrupting meetings, the team might not be open with me or might not let me sit in their meetings. I think I can do more good on a larger scale by watch-ing the team with as little interference as possible from me and using my research findings to influence future teams' behaviors."

I look at Ken's face. He doesn't seem convinced.

"Besides," I continue, "there are therapists and professionals on the team, and I might derail plans they have, things they are working toward, if I interrupt. One of the key concepts of systems of care is to empower the families. If I jump in to stand up for them, won't that disempower them?" Ken is nodding, so I relax a little as we move on to the next question.

Research Methodology

"Cris," Carolyn interjects. "Could you explain your methodology?"

"I'll be taking a case study approach to this research. As Jarrett [1992] says, a case study is a 'detailed and in-depth investigation of a single unit' [p. 176], and my unit of measurement will be one community mental health system of care child and family team. I'll study them in detail and complexity."

"Could you discuss your data collection methods?" Carolyn asks.

"I'll observe many different kinds of team interactions, and I'll listen to the way team members talk about, and with, their other team members. Therefore, I'll be using a number of approaches to the data collection, which lets me, as Richardson [2000] said, crystallize the data. Crystallization recognizes that reality is multidimensional, deep, and complex and that understanding a phenomenon requires several different approaches to the research investigation. Crystallization will contribute to my research rigor by allowing me to immerse myself in the experience from many different perspectives [Lincoln & Guba, 1985; Patton, 2002; Stake, 1995]. I plan to conduct in-depth interviews with all team members, observe all team meetings and interactions—other than therapy sessions—between team members and the family, and conduct three interactive focus groups with the family and team."

Art sits forward and changes the subject. "Cris, tell us about the narrative approach that you'll be using to write up your research."

I nod. "I plan to use narrative ethnography, which is an intimate, more vulnerable form of writing and researching. I'll be using a narrative approach to my analysis that will let me think through the stories as I write them. Thinking with and through narratives help us to make sense of our research [Bochner, Ellis, & Tillman-Healy, 1998; Coles, 1989; Frank, 1995; Nelson, 2001; Polkinghorne, 1988; Skjorshammer, 2002]. Narrative understanding helps us to see the story's significance within the larger community [Nelson, 1998]. We live our lives in stories, and we talk in stories, and we have an innate disposition to think in stories" [Bruner, 1990; Mortola & Carlson, 2003].

"What will your final product be like?" asks Art.

"I'll write evocative narratives that will link my personal experiences with my ethnographic insights [Ellis & Bochner, 2000; Reed-Danahay, 2001; Tedlock, 2000]. I'll use a narrative writing approach that will bring together narratives from the team's point of view; narratives from my point of view as researcher; and autoethnographic and reflexive narratives on my personal reflections on issues raised in the course of doing the research. Some details will be fictional, or imaginary, but the voices will reflect the voices of participants. The resulting product will be an evocative narrative, reminiscent of a novel, with characters, plot, action, and movement."

"What are the ethics of writing a story about your research?" Carolyn asks.

"Well," I respond thoughtfully. "I will, of course, alter names and details to protect the anonymity and confidentiality of the participants. Of course, taking some creative license with some details will also let me create a coherent narrative out of many different observations and interviews. So, I'll change the names and identifying details in this story, and I'll combine interview quotes from some participants with those of other participants. Throughout my writing, I will always attempt to stay close to the truth, nature, and character of the experiences as they are told to me and as I experience and understand them."

"Cris, I'm sure I've never seen research that looks like that in my field," Bob says with a smile. "It sounds as though it will be a unique study and fascinating perspective. I think it will make great and useful reading for many of us in the field."

I smile at him. "I sure hope so."

CHAPTER 2

R. M. S. Titanic: Meeting Poverty and Disability Face to Face

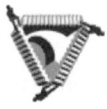

The room is pitch-black. The stage lights are slowly turned up so that the room is dimly lit. Smoke gradually fills the stage, then the theater. The smell of burned ash penetrates the air. The stage curtains are torn and dark with soot.

In the background, a sign reads: "R. M. S. Titanic."

Suddenly, the spotlight in the center of the stage is turned up just enough so that I can be seen. My clothes are blackened. I am alone.

Behind me, portholes illuminate. Past the portholes are green neon signs. One at a time, they light up and begin blinking, until they all are blinking messages:

> *Cleanliness is next to Godliness.*
> *The Lord helps those who help themselves.*
> *Early to bed, and early to rise, makes a man healthy, wealthy, and wise.*
> *The early bird gets the worm.*
> *Make hay while the sun shines.*
> *Vessels large may venture more, but little boats should keep near shore.*

The boom of thunder pierces the silence, and lightning flashes.

I look down at the ground. Water is rising. It is up to my ankles. I pick up a small bucket and begin bailing. The water continues to rise.

I bail water.

The water is up to my calves.

I bail water.

The water is up to my knees.

I bail water.

The water is up to my hips.

CRIS: Help! Help me! I need help!

The rear of the stage is lit, and people can be seen on shore.

PERSON 1: Keep working! You're doing fine! Remember, you have strengths!

PERSON 2: Work harder! Work harder!

PERSON 3: (*Holds up papers*) You need to fill out this paperwork!

PERSON 2: You shouldn't have gone out in the water in that boat!

PERSON 1: We're here to help! Call us if you need anything!

PERSON 3: I have a family support plan for you! You need to sign the paperwork!

The sound of the thunder gets louder. The voices get louder, repeating their lines, all at the same time. Crashes of lightning become more frequent. Smoke continues to pour in, and the neon lights continue to blink.

I bail water.

The water is up to my neck.

FADE TO BLACK.

Poverty Sucks

I am at work, and Alan, the Executive Director of the Center for Children and Families, calls. They have a family for my case study.

"This family is one of Nancy's," Alan explains. "They're a real interesting case."

"Tell me about them."

"We just started working with them. It's a really poor family with three kids. The father has health issues. They're going to be involved in a lot of different systems: mental health, education, maybe recreation or social, primary health, financial. The kid is just getting to a point where he's not going to be successful at his high school. In middle school, they really had much more control over the teachers' reactions to the kids. They had the ability to remove the kids from the classroom and settle them down. They could de-escalate situations, and that worked real well with him in the middle school. So he's been bounced out of two high schools and has just been put in Washington High, which is an ESE—Exceptional Student Education—and SED school. I just recently met the family. We went out and spent a Friday morning with Mom and Dad."

"Hmmm, what are they like?"

"It's an interesting kind of situation. This is a family that has extreme issues of poverty. They're disorganized, they collect everything. They have medical issues along with some psychiatric issues, and some family issues relating to, again, extreme poverty. The kid has had years and years of actual clinical intervention, with a diagnosis of ADHD. But I'm wondering whether this is an accurate diagnosis or not. The family is very willing to participate. It's probably been five or six years since I've been in a home environment that's this severe and depressed and oriented toward poverty."

"Wow!" I comment.

"It's a very severe environment," he reiterates.

"In what way?" I wonder what I'm in for.

"The home is almost ready to be condemned. It's in shambles. They pretty much collect everything and keep it."

I take a deep breath. "That certainly sounds interesting. I'd love to work with Nancy. I'm game if you think they would be good for my research," I say.

"They're very poor," Alan reiterates. "Their poverty will be a huge factor in their services."

"When can I meet them?"

I'm curious about how our society constructs poverty, so I do some reading. The Puritan, Calvinist, and Baptist religious movements of the seventeenth century introduced the notion that the distribution of material goods was a gift from God, and, thus, wealth was a sign of God's blessing. The converse thus became a cultural belief—that poverty is a curse from God (Weber, 2003). Although most U.S. Americans say they believe in equality, most people in our society also believe that competence should be rewarded by success and incompetence should be rewarded by failure (Jencks et al., 2003). These two ideas together introduce a moral dimension to the issue of poverty in our culture—that poor people are somehow deserving of their poverty and thus deserve an inferior status as a result.

Poverty is an interesting construct, however. Poverty has been said to be a "vague concept" (Sen, 1992, p. 48) because it is typically defined in relative rather than absolute terms. In our culture, we usually define poverty as being about half of what the average American family makes (and below) (Jencks et al., 2003). This definition is striking when we realize that this half is much more than most people made just 30 years ago, measured in today's dollars. As a result, it's easy to see that income does not reflect the ability to purchase goods or services but rather reflects the cost of participating in a social system. People who make less than "normal" in our society are accordingly excluded from society (Jencks et al., 2003). People who are "core poor" (Clark & Qizilbash, 2008, p. 519) are people for whom—based on their needs and capabilities—there is no doubt that they are poor. But being "core poor" is about more than a lack of access. These extremely poor people may have a hard time *accepting* their lack of access and have an especially strong desire to obtain services, such as healthcare services, most acutely when their peer group has a deficit in those services (Barr & Clark, 2010). In addition, because earning a living in our society now requires high levels of competence and education compared to past generations, the array of ways in which a person can participate in our social system is much narrower today than in the past and has a great deal to do with ability and disability. For example, people with disabilities suffer from earnings deficits of 21 percent to over 50 percent compared to people without disabilities (Brown & Emery, 2010), and during the recent recession people with disabilities have been laid off from their jobs disproportionally more than people without disabilities (Kaye, 2010). In addition, competence today depends more on one's personality than one's skills, a clear disadvantage for people with mental, emotional, and behavioral disabilities (Jencks et al., 2003). Poverty is also problematic for parents and families, because our culture believes that money is important to be a "good parent." Money purchases necessities (food and medical care) and lets parents spend more time with their children. Because it is believed that children respond to their environment, an environment of poverty is believed to set a child up for a lack of success as they grow up. Behaviors that might be thought of as a rational response to poverty are often viewed as dysfunctional in our larger culture and sometimes result in the interference of child welfare or other social authorities in the family's life (Mayer, 2003). Poverty sucks, in so many ways, I think.

I think about how today's American family struggles against an ideal of unrealistic expectations imposed by our culture. They're fighting a losing battle. Family times are now performances of family—and even much more so when enacted in public settings (Gillis, 1996). Therefore, whether or not a person is a "good-enough parent" has to do with the nature of our understandings of the relationships between people and objects. If our ideas about reality are socially constructed—which I believe they are—it stands to reason, then, that deviance, which is based firmly on our construction of reality, is also socially constructed. All of us live within our illusions. Where is the point at which illusions cross the line from normal to abnormal? I think that this is a very important point, and one that is not taken into account often enough, especially within governmental organizations charged to determine when a family is a "good-enough" family—such as when the child welfare system determines whether to reunify a family or remove a child from their home. The lines seem to be one of a matter of degree. Perhaps all families have traces of deviance while all families also have traces of normality (Henry, 1965; Hoffman, 1981). If poverty and parenting can be thought of as social constructions, behaviors that might seem dysfunctional at first look might actually be a rational response to poverty or other situations in which a family finds itself.

The Initial Meeting

A week later, Nancy's voice is on my voice mail. "Cris," she says, "I know you haven't had a chance to meet the Stewarts yet, but we're having a team meeting in the morning. At the school. There's an emergency situation, and we couldn't wait. I hope you can come."

My mind races. Of course—I'll make sure I can come. This is the family I'm going to be working with in my research. I begin making a list, pushing aside the regret that I hadn't had a chance to meet the family before the team meeting. Okay, now, what do I need to do? Make plenty of copies of the informed consent forms. Make sure Nancy gives me a chance to explain my research before she begins the meeting. Oh, and, find out where the school is! I go to the MapQuest web page as I clear a stack of papers from my desk. Won't get back to that project today. I wonder what time in the morning the meeting is. I look up Nancy's number to call her and ask.

Despite numerous phone messages, I do not hear back from Nancy. I remember a comment she made the week before and guess that the meeting will be at 9:00 A.M. at Washington High. I hope I'm right.

With little difficulty I find the school from the MapQuest directions. It's a picture of poverty itself. Standing as a barrier between a once comfortable residential neighborhood and the urban interchange of two major interstate highways dwarfing the buildings below, it's small and dingy, with peeling paint and barbed wire twisted along its perimeter walls. The bulk of the school grounds consist of trailer-classrooms (euphemistically called "portables," as if they are going to be moved, as if they are not permanent structures in this throw-away school with society's throw-away children).

I check in at the office, obediently following signs instructing "All Visitors Must Report to Office." When Nancy walks in, I am relieved to see her.

"Hi, I was hoping I guessed right!" I say, trying not to sound scolding.

"I'm so sorry I didn't call you back," she responds. "I was in meetings. I'm glad you're here!" she adds as she squeezes my hand.

The meeting is in a large classroom that, when it's not being used for meetings, is the time-out room for children with behavioral problems. As they arrive, I greet the team members and explain my research. Warren, a dark man with a large athletic build and strong handshake, works in the school system but is here as informal support for the family. Jane, the SED specialist for the school, has short brown hair and is dressed in practical shoes and a denim jumper. Peggy, the school social worker, is dressed like a therapist and smiles warmly at me. Mr. Camelini, the SED teacher with graying hair and a worried frown, arrives last. I meet the parents—Mr. and Mrs. Stewart, the mother and step-father. Mrs. Stewart is a small woman. I'm barely 5′3″, and she's several inches shorter than I am. She's dressed in blue jeans and a T-shirt, and is very thin, probably about my age. Her long brown hair hangs down her back. Mr. Stewart, also in jeans and a T-shirt, with unruly brown hair touched with gray, is in a wheelchair (multiple sclerosis, I remember Nancy telling me). He has a nice smile as I greet him. After I get the consent forms signed, I take a seat in a student desk, slightly away from the table, as I begin to take notes.

Nancy begins the meeting. "We're going to start with strengths. I personally have seen Kevin's strengths. Kevin is smart and loving." She reads from a stack of notes in front of her. "Mr. Stewart is interested, caring, and concerned. Mrs. Stewart's main strength is follow-through. It was hard for them to get here because of transportation problems, but they're here—on time," she points out. "She follows through. She's made the initial neurological appointment for Kevin."

Nancy turns to Warren. "What would you say the strengths of Kevin are?"

Warren doesn't hesitate. "I've known Kevin since the 6th grade. He loves to read. You need to find books he loves to read," he suggests to the teacher. "He has a high level of reading skills; he's a good speller. He has a high functioning vocabulary." He pauses and looks around the table. "Sometimes, he goes AWOL. He needs time to himself. I'd just give him a book to give him time to get himself together to be able to go back to class."

Warren's suggestion is interrupted by the intercom. "Mrs. Little, Mrs. Little. Kevin Stewart has left his classroom." As Jane runs out the door, the intercom sounds again. "The school resource officer has him."

I take notes as a drama unfolds. Screaming can be heard outside the door. Mrs. Stewart runs out into the courtyard and returns with a screaming, thrashing young boy. Kevin is 14 years old but looks about eight. Even then, he would be the skinniest 8-year-old I have ever seen. His sandy-colored hair is wild, and he is out of control. He runs into the room, screaming, rapidly circling the room, knocking over chairs, running into the table, tossing chairs out of his way as he runs. When he runs into the back corner of the room, Mrs. Stewart goes after him. "I know how to handle him," she says as she glances back to the group.

A man dressed in a police uniform enters the room, followed by Jane. Warren greets him like an old friend. "It's okay," he tells him. "He'll be okay." Turning to the group, he says, "he knows we're meeting in here, talking about him. The last time we did that, at the other school, he was moved to a new school. He doesn't like change."

The officer sits down at the desk and picks up a magazine, nonchalantly reading it while remaining alert to the drama in the room.

Mrs. Stewart and Kevin are in the corner, arguing.

Nancy, trying to restart the meeting, hands Warren a piece of paper. "This is the situation," she begins to explain.

Warren interjects. "It sounds like a typical situation. He went back to class. The kids were poking at him, making fun of him. That always sets him off."

Mr. Camelini hands me a piece of paper. "It's a checklist of strengths," he explains. I nod as the yelling between Kevin and his mom gets closer to us. She smacks him on his arm as they rush outside. The officer follows.

"Why don't we continue?" Nancy suggests.

"Should we be having the meeting without Mom?" Jane asks, a concerned look on her face.

Nancy nods. "We're in a time crunch. We have her permission."

Peggy turns to Mr. Stewart. "Are you okay with telling her what we said?" she asks.

He nods.

"Kevin needs a place where he can go," Mr. Camelini suggests.

"We're shorthanded right now. There's no one in timeout," Jane responds.

Warren leans forward. "What worked before, when he had a problem in class, he would come into our program office. We'd put him at a desk where he could read."

Jane shakes her head. "We tried that yesterday. He kept running in and out."

Warren continues, as if she hadn't interrupted him. "He would sit and read. We'd give him a cracker if he was hungry." Warren looks around the table and sees that he has everyone's attention, so he continues. "Kevin had the fourth lunch. Since he was up at 6:00 A.M., by the time lunch came, it was six hours after breakfast, and he'd become hungry. I'd invite him to come to my office. I had a refrigerator, I had juice. He'd come in and sit down. That would stabilize him."

Mrs. Stewart comes back in with Kevin, who still looks angry. Sitting down next to her, he folds his arms and sullenly looks straight ahead. He kicks his chair with his foot, loudly.

Jane turns to Kevin, "Would you like to sit in time-out?"

"You can read," Mrs. Stewart offers.

Kevin doesn't respond, and Peggy turns to Mr. Camelini. "How many kids do you have in your classroom?"

"Nine." He explains Kevin's progress to her. "In a few minutes, once he gets himself together, you'll see a well-mannered boy."

Jane nods. "Oh, I've seen that. He's even taken responsibility for his problems."

"Oh, yes," Mr. Camelini agrees. "He needs something to read, something to get his interest. In a few minutes, he'll be able to see where he went wrong. Kevin needs to understand that when he went out and interrupted, it was the officer's job to protect him. Interventions would help him a lot better if we could bring him in here so he could slow himself down. Once he's able to gather his thoughts, he's powerful."

Jane frowns. "He used to be able to, but now he's on a downward spiral. It's not working anymore."

Peggy interjects. "We initially had very poor interactions with each other. We've explored the issues from yesterday." I notice that she is talking to Mr. Camelini, yet looking at Kevin from time to time as she speaks. Mrs. Stewart and Kevin are having a side conversation during this discussion. They seem to be arguing about his sitting still during the meeting.

"Yesterday," Jane adds, "Kevin had an altercation with another youth. I told him that we need to work on both sides, there are two sides. He wanted sympathy from me, but I was also trying to get him to see his responsibility in what was going on."

I make a mental note of the deficit-strength tension in the meeting. This happens quite a bit in team meetings, especially the first meeting, since staying in strengths mode while dealing with concrete problems is quite a challenge.

Nancy turns to Kevin. "Mr. Camelini says you can accept responsibility, you're friendly. You have a high reading level, you have a large vocabulary. You're capable of controlling your behavior, and you want to do right. I know you know what's okay and what's not okay. We're a team of people who care about you. That's why we're meeting—to talk about helping you."

Now I notice how Nancy artfully accomplishes two things—turns the discussion back to strengths and "humanizes" Kevin by talking to him rather than talking about him.

Peggy interjects. "Let's talk about how we can proceed. Here, you don't go to time-out unless someone tells you to go to time-out. At his other school, he could ask to go to time-out—before he got upset," she explains. "My point is, time-out could be a positive thing, as opposed to punishment."

Mr. Camelini agrees. "He'd be able to gather himself together." He pauses. "The officer seems to set him off."

Peggy nods and turns to Nancy and Mr. and Mrs. Stewart. "The officer touched him. The minute he was touched by him, he went off. He started calling him lots of names. The officer couldn't let go of him, it was a safety issue. It was a respect issue. He hit the officer. The officer could have cuffed him."

I think to myself how they now have moved beyond blaming Kevin for his problems to understanding the social and environmental context of what is going on.

The arguing between Kevin and Mrs. Stewart at the corner of the table gets louder.

"No!" Kevin yells. "I won't go!"

"Kevin," Mrs. Stewart responds in a loud voice, "you have to do what we say!"

Nancy turns to them, and addresses Kevin. "Kevin, you need to hear this." Kevin looks up.

Warren turns to Kevin. "Kevin, I know this officer very well. He has never hurt a kid. If you listen to him, he won't put his hands on you. If you do not comply with him, he has to take action. It's not anything against you. If you listen, you will never have a problem with him." Kevin responds with head nods and shrugs. He says nothing.

Mrs. Stewart turns to Jane. "See, this is what I go through."

Kevin and Mr. Stewart argue about whether Kevin is old enough to be arrested. Warren enters the conversation and addresses Kevin. "There are kids younger than you in jail."

Nancy addresses Kevin. "Listen to him. This man cares about you."

Kevin leaves his chair and stands next to Warren. When he puts his arm around Warren's shoulder, Warren responds by putting his arm around Kevin's waist. After they speak quietly, Kevin leaves the room.

Mrs. Stewart speaks to the group. "You saw how I had to restrain him. This is what I have to do at home."

No one responds to Mrs. Stewart's comment. Nancy tries to bring the meeting back to order. Mr. Camelini begins his report again. "He has higher functioning than the other students. But he rushes through his work so he can play. Letting him out to do reading, that's a good idea, a good intervention. Letting him out for safety value, that's a good idea." He adjusts his glasses and continues. "The classroom is more structured, so he does better in there than in P.E. or computer class. Kevin does say bad, racial things, and he threatens the other kids. And, he's the smallest kid in class."

I remember this is why Nancy thinks his problem is neurological. Threatening kids over twice your size is an indication of a disconnect between behavior and consequence, she thinks.

Peggy nods. "They show great restraint. They know where he's coming from."

Warren turns to Mr. Camelini. "I'd like to talk to your classroom. I'd like to commend them on their restraint. They need to be reinforced as African-American males. They need to be confirmed, that they're on the right track. In my work, I give interventions with young people to tell them that there are other ways, you don't have to react. I can teach positive anger management skills."

Nancy smiles. "That sounds very positive."

Peggy asks, "Can we do something to lower the frequency of him saying those things? He craves attention. If they ignore him, it'll escalate."

Warren shakes his head. "If I teach his classmates to defuse it, to say to him, 'I see you're upset. Tell me why you're upset,' it will get them to think on a higher level. I'll teach them not to personally absorb his anger."

"That's great," Peggy responds, "but where does Kevin learn to change his behaviors? We need to give him some sort of tools so he's not doing it so often."

"If we change his community, change the way they react to him, it will change his thought process," Warren answers. "They'll be a community in a different way altogether. Now they're pushing him. Instead, community could become something positive. We'll get the kids to role play and interact. Get them to think entirely differently working for each other rather than against each other. We can change his entire situation."

This is systems theory in action, I think to myself. Systems theory suggests that changing one thing in the environment will change the entire environment.

"When will you start?" Peggy asks.

"Right away, as soon as it's okay with Mr. Camelini."

"I can arrange anything."

Nancy smiles. "This is an extremely positive, concrete way we can move forward. I want to stay positive. But, to stay positive, we have to keep him in school. He's been having problems on the bus. His parents can't transport him. He needs to stay on the bus, he needs to stay safe."

"The bus," Jane adds to the story. "This is the reason we're meeting today. There was an incident yesterday. He yelled racial slurs out the window to the kids standing on the street. To a bunch of street thugs. They responded by trying to get on the bus. The bus driver drove off, and Kevin grabbed at her ankles while she was driving, evidently to try to stop her. The bus drivers' instructions in a situation like that are to pull over and call the police. She didn't. But she could have. She's also bending over backward with him."

"We need to talk with the bus driver. We've got to set up some sort of plan," Nancy suggests.

"Kevin won't tell us the truth," Mrs. Stewart adds. "We have to find out from others what happened."

"We can brainstorm as adults," Nancy says.

"I hope you all can. I can't," Mrs. Stewart responds in frustration.

Warren interjects. "Where does the aide sit? The aide should sit in the seat with him. They should become best buddies. I know some other kids on his bus; I'll get one of them to handle the back of the bus. I can engage the other kids in the process. Kevin needs to have his own seat. He needs to be with an aide."

"The aide is for the whole bus," Mr. Camelini explains.

"Can we request an individual aide for Kevin?" Nancy asks. "We need to approach transportation before they approach us. Ask for this help. We need to tell them we're working on it. We need to make a proactive approach."

Peggy asks, "Will the bus supervisor have a copy of the report? This may be a whole new thing we have to deal with."

Nancy nods. "We need to approach them before they approach us. Who should ask for a one-on-one aide?"

Jane explains the process. "It's very hard with the budget situation. There are bus shortages, driver shortages."

"We'll write a letter from our agency. Maybe that will help," Nancy offers.

Mrs. Stewart leans toward Nancy. "Can I talk to you outside?" They step out of the room.

Nancy returns and explains. "Mr. and Mrs. Stewart need to leave. They're taking the bus home and have to be home when their other two kids get home from school. We'll put in a request to pay for a taxi home next time," she offers.

Nancy quickly reviews the meeting. "Warren will do an intervention with the class. We'll ask for an aide on the bus." She turns to Mrs. Stewart. "Can you ask his therapist to do a home assessment?"

Mrs. Stewart's face gets red and her voice is loud. She explodes. "I asked. She refused. We have been asking for help. No one will listen."

"What if we ask someone else?" Nancy asks.

Mrs. Stewart responds, loudly. "Anything else Kevin needs, he'll get, whatever it takes."

"We're going to enforce the time-out," Jane suggests.

"He can get food and books," Nancy reminds her.

Mr. Camelini leans forward. "We should really excuse him from P.E. Those kids are rough. Those kids are too big for him. Any unstructured time, he has trouble with."

Nancy leans forward. "Can the time-out person understand she's not rewarding negative behavior for letting him read; it's a way to calm him?"

"Can I make a suggestion? He likes to draw," suggests Mrs. Stewart.

Mr. Camelini nods at her. "I can get him a marker, and a book on how to draw."

After Mr. and Mrs. Stewart leave, the group remains around the table for a few more minutes.

"We didn't get to discuss the condition of their house," adds Peggy.

"It needs to be cleaned," Nancy agrees. "But, we have to be respectful."

As I drive home, I think back about the meeting. What a soap opera! What about the emotional outburst from Kevin—what was the trigger? What functions in this system did the outburst serve? Was he asking for voice? Was he expressing pain? What are the patterns that keep us locked into these ways of communicating?

We can't escape our family history. What functions do disabilities play in a family? How does a family communicate through illness (Hoffman, 1981; Minuchin, 1993)? At times of change, patterns have to be renegotiated and recreated (Minuchin, 1993). What patterns is this family creating and recreating? How is the team influencing their patterns? Systems theorists suggest that irrational behavior in a family is required in order for the family to maintain equilibrium, or balance (Hoffman, 1981). How does this system lock the family into using illness as communication, and what are they communicating?

Help Him

Today there's a person with a sign asking for money at the end of my off-ramp. There used to be lots of people begging for money; we live near a truck stop, and hitchhikers from the north stop there on their way to warmer climates. I haven't seen any in a while—probably too cold this time of year for a lot of travelers. I drive by him, trying not to meet his eyes, feeling guilty for doing so. I say a quick prayer for him: "Lord, please help him." I get a strong answer back: "No, I sent YOU to help him!" Whether this is actually a voice from God or not, I don't know, but it sure gets both my attention and my conscience! I feel weighted down by guilt the rest of the day.

Another World

A week later, I am in my year-old Honda Accord, late as usual, driving to my interview with Mr. and Mrs. Stewart. I'm following the directions closely. Mrs. Stewart is a very good direction-giver, which is a good thing, because I can get lost very easily, and this is an unfamiliar part of town. It's as if I'm transported into another world from the urban city I usually see in the parts of town I frequent. I pass a Cattleman's Livestock Market. A sign advertises a sale every Monday. A hair and barber shop. A used-auto sales lot. Two bondsmen. A wholesale auto auction. I pass a big Budweiser truck. A Circle K. A couple of warehouses. A construction company. Some dirt roads. An auto body shop. A church—"The Holy Church of Christ." Its front façade is made up of some kind of a fake stone. A pawn shop—fast and easy cash for anything of value.

The Stewarts live on a mostly tree-lined, quiet residential street off the industrial street. Cars and trucks race by less than a block away, yet their street has rows of modest homes behind chain-link fenced yards with patches of grass and dirt and leaves. The houses have white siding, maybe what you'd call clapboard. There are a couple of For Sale signs on the street. This morning there are full garbage cans standing along the road.

I pull up to their house and try to decide where to park. I try to avoid parking in front of their trash can, but their yard is so narrow, it is hard to park in front of their house without also parking in front of a neighbor's house. Their house has no grass, not a blade of it; it's all dirt. And clutter. Their yard is strewn with what looks like junk—rusting metal furniture lying on its side, children's toys.

I notice that the side of their house, up to about 7 feet, is newly painted white. Above that is peeling, very badly peeling, faded white paint. To get inside, I walk up a very steep wooden ramp. I feel like I'm climbing into a fortress. I momentarily slip going up the ramp, and I grab onto the door frame to catch myself. I am in a tiny screen porch. I step through papers and junk on the floor, find their front door, and knock.

"Come on in!" a voice inside responds to my knock. As I open the door, my eyes have to adjust to the darkness. The windows are covered with what looks like very dirty sheets. The walls are black with dust.

There's stuff all over the floor, and I walk along a pathway through the room, the only clear space on the floor. The sensation is of being in a very dirty and dusty cave, foggy from their cigarette smoke. My nostrils take in the acrid smell of smoke, and I stifle a sneeze. Within seconds, I feel a layer of some sort of dirt or slime covering my teeth and skin. I ignore the growls of their dog and try not to notice the roach crawling across the floor.

I locate Mrs. Stewart in the fog and sit down on their living room couch as I greet her. The couch is also blackened with dirt, and wish I hadn't worn my white pants today. Their dog comes over for a sniff. I recognize its breed—a miniature pincher. We just had our miniature pincher put to sleep a few months ago. Their dog is adorable and quite affectionate now that he has figured out that I must be friendly.

I notice the embroidery on the walls. "How beautiful," I say.

Mrs. Stewart comments, smiling at my noticing. "This is one thing I'm good at."

I notice another wall hanging. "Did you paint that? Or stencil it?"

"I painted it," she responds proudly.

I'm impressed. I think of my mom, who had strong sewing, art, and craft skills. She spent our childhoods decorating our house with her beautifully constructed crafts. This is where the similarity ends, though. Appearance was very important to Mom. Too important, I often thought. Our large and spacious house was always spotless. We had a lower-middle-class income but lived within an upper-middle-class means. Borrowing money and pinching pennies was one of our family's secrets.

My thoughts momentary go back to a scene from my childhood. I am 12 years old. My dad and I are in the living room, relaxing while we eat ice cream in from of the TV. Suddenly, there is a loud crash in the kitchen, followed by yelling and cursing, and another crash. Mom is throwing things. I make out a few words, something about "dirty house!"

Dad's face pales. "Go help your mother," he instructs. I get up, hesitantly. I know that I shouldn't leave my ice cream bowl in the living room, but I'm sufficiently afraid of Mom's temper to stay out of the kitchen. I decide to take it upstairs with me, where it will be out of her sight for a while, maybe until she calms down. I fight the anger creeping up my neck. "It's not fair!" I say to myself. "Other mothers don't have temper tantrums! If she wanted us to do something, why didn't she just ask us?" I go up to my room, resisting the urge to stomp. Staying below the radar is a good idea when she gets like this.

Resentment washes over me. My older sister has a disability, and my younger sister is "the baby." It seems to me that I end up doing the bulk of the housework. "It's not fair!" I think again. I pull the vacuum cleaner from the hall closet. Our clean house hides our dirty secrets—emotional problems, money problems, health problems. I'm the good girl in our family. Good girls keep things clean.

My attention returns to Mrs. Stewart's wall. "Is that fabric art?" I admire. "You are good!"

"My mother taught me how," she explains.

I sigh. "My mother tried to teach me, but I didn't have the patience to learn from her. She was very disappointed. You could make a lot of money selling stuff like that," I observe.

"If I had room to do it, I could, but as you can see, the house is so small," she responds.

" 'Cause you've got three kids, right?" I respond, trying to smoothly turn the conversation into the direction of my interview questions. "It is small for three kids," I agree. "Tell me a little bit about your family, just some background for me. You've got three kids," I begin again.

"The three youngest are at home," she explains. "Kevin is 14, Karla is 13, and Gary is 11."

I note her reference to their being the three youngest and remember that Nancy had mentioned she had an earlier family removed from her home. I hope she's not offended by my asking about them. "These are the three at home. You have some kids"—I trail off to let her finish my sentence.

"Six others," she explains.

"They're older, not at home anymore?" I clarify.

"Yes," she verifies. I leave the story at that until she decides to self-disclose more.

I turn to Mr. Stewart. "You're their step-father, correct? I'm a step-mother myself, so I'd be interested in your opinions of what it's like." He doesn't respond to my attempt at rapport, so I move on to my next question. "Tell me a little bit about Kevin. What has caused you to seek services?"

"He's ADHD. It's the violent tendency that we really need help with," Mrs. Stewart explains. "Kevin was diagnosed with ADHD when he was in kindergarten. They had EMH—Emotionally Mentally Handicapped— teachers. Then, his school lost the funding for that, and he had to transfer to Oak Park. That's where he was until he went to Franklin, so he's been ADHD from Day One."

"Why did you contact the Center for Children and Families?" I ask.

"Actually it was the school that did. When Kevin got into Washington High he was doing okay for a couple weeks, and then all of a sudden he changed, and he started becoming violent. The violence is the main thing we're concerned with. I mean Kevin's smart."

"He's very engaging," I add. "So that violence is a new behavior."

"Yes, very new. It frightens me."

"What is the Center for Children and Families doing for you?"

"So far they've helped us to get paint for the outside of the house. I've already got part of it painted, but I haven't been able to do very much." She nods toward her husband. "He can't do much, so I do most of it."

"Sure," I acknowledge. She's got more energy than I do; I'd never consider painting my house if I could help it. I think back to 20 years ago when my husband Jerry and I renovated a house. After that, we'd always said we'd hire somebody to do the work next time. "So they've helped you with paint. What else have they helped you with?"

"They've helped us with Kevin," Mrs. Stewart responds.

"They've helped us with Kevin, too." Mr. Stewart repeats. I realize that this is the first thing he has said during the interview.

"What have they done with Kevin?"

"Except for what they do at the school, I don't know what else they've done, really. Other than actually visiting Kevin, having one-on-one sessions with Kevin at the school, which they do," Mrs. Stewart responds thoughtfully.

"Nancy does that?" I ask.

Mrs. Stewart nods. "Nancy was supposed to be here today, but she was supposed to call first, and she didn't call. So I don't know. She might not make it. I've been trying to get her to see if she can get us a new bathtub, 'cause he's fixed our old one twice already. It's got this gigantic crack in it. I'm not worried about me falling. I can live with that. But I'm worried about him or one of the kids. All we need is the money in hand. We can fix it ourselves. We can get one from the flea market."

"Thinking of your whole team, tell me a story of a typical interaction that you have with them."

"Other than the meetings, we usually don't see them."

"What's Nancy coming out this morning for?"

"She just wants to work on our assistance budget. We've been doing some checking, and I found a lot of homes. Maybe if we could get enough money to pay this place off, we could either use this as a down payment or just sell it and be able to put that money toward one of them government homes."

Mr. Stewart adds to her answer. "See, this house is good for two people. It's small. See all that, from that door on back was added on. It was only a two-bedroom cottage-type."

I look around. From my vantage point in the living room, it appears that I can see the entire house. "So what you've got here is the living room/ dining room, then you've got the kitchen, then that's a bedroom?"

They both nod. "There's two bedrooms and a bathroom. There's no storage. We don't have any closet except the one in our room." I think of how all of our closets in our house are full, and we don't have any kids at home. I wonder how a person can live with no closets. No wonder their house is so cluttered.

I continue with my interview. "So, how does Nancy treat you? What is Nancy like with you?"

"Most of the time she treats us pretty good, but once in a while she gets—maybe she got stressed out or something but she's just—she's a little edgy," Mrs. Stewart responds in a confidential tone.

Mr. Stewart echoes her response. "She gets a little edgy."

I nod. "Give me an example." Nancy's always seemed very calm to me. I wonder what it would take to make her edgy.

"When I was trying to talk to her about maybe using some of that home improvement budget to get a new bathtub, she practically bit my head off."

"What did she say?"

"She said, 'it's not for that.' And I'm thinking, 'if it's for home improvement, wouldn't a brand new bathtub come under that heading?' I mean, I didn't say it because I didn't want to get my head bit off. I'll be honest with you. I do have a bad temper. I've learned over the past 20 some-odd years to control it. So if you get on my bad side, God help you, because I'll put it bluntly, I can be a bitch." I wonder if that comment is also a warning directed at me. I make a mental note to try not to get on her bad side. I focus my attention back on her explanation of their attempts to fix up their house.

"We applied for programs to help us with this house, but every program we applied for, they called us back and said they had run out of funds. We had one of the programs set up for a grant to replace the windows and put in central air. Six months later they called us and said they had run out of funds."

Mr. Stewart jumps in. "Then they say, when we get our new fiscal budget, you're top of the list. Fiscal budget comes, we don't hear nothing."

Mrs. Stewart nods and Mr. Stewart continues his story. "It took us six years to get a roof on this place. My dad finally was able to buy the supplies, then we got help through a church."

"No, it was from the city, it had the teenagers," Mrs. Stewart corrects him.

"Yeah, but they worked for the church," Mr. Stewart reiterated. "But other than that, that's the only program that's ever done anything. This house has aluminum siding on the outside that we put on. We stripped it off of a trailer, and we installed it ourselves. With the MS now, I can't finish it." I nod, and he continues to explain. "I've been disabled since '78. I was born with a hole in my heart. Blind in one eye, brittle bones. So I've been in and out of the hospital all my life. And in '78 I got hit by a tractor trailer. I was in the hospital for a year and a half. That was my second accident."

I raise my eyebrows. "You're a walking miracle!" He chuckles at the comment.

I move us back to our interview questions. I'm trying to listen for stories of interactions with team members. I'm a little dismayed that they don't have any. I wonder if the team knows as much about the family as I do from talking to them for 30 minutes in their home. "Tell me about the team meeting. I would really love to know what you think about the team meeting."

"It gives us a chance to hear what's going on at school, and also to make it known how he behaves at home."

Mr. Stewart nods. "Focusing on education is very good for Kevin."

"Why do you say that?"

"Because education is good for everybody, and the more Kevin learns, the easier it will be for him to ease into a stable life. But the one thing they don't really want to address is the incidents of violence. I don't know why. I know there ain't much they can do about his behavior at home, but when we try to explain to them, it's like they don't care. But they should care. Because what happens at home could carry over into the school day." Mrs. Stewart's voice is loud and animated. "We're afraid he's going to hurt somebody."

Mr. Stewart joins in the story. "He'll tell her to shut up and leave him alone, and he'll go in there and slam the door, hit his head on the floor, on the wall."

"One minute Kevin can be a sweet as can be, and the next minute he's in your face, calling you a bitch, all kind of names," Mrs. Stewart adds. "He says he hates us. I've got to where it hurts, but I don't let it bother me anymore. Like this morning, Gary didn't say nothing to him, but Kevin hauled off and punched him. For nothing."

I observe, "What a way to start your day." My mom and I had a very stormy relationship during my teenage years. I wonder how she would have described it to an outsider. At least I never hit anyone. I push away the memory of my mom slapping me.

"Exactly. I'll be truthful. My home life, when I was growing up, it wasn't the worst and it wasn't the best. It was average for the times. So I can take a lot of punishment, and my first ex-husband was real abusive. I can handle pretty much anything." She nods toward Mr. Stewart. "What

I am worried about is him and Kevin and Gary. I'm worried about Kevin hurting himself."

Mr. Stewart adds, "Here lately he's been threatening to get scissors, knives, and hurt himself."

"Us too. He was going to take a knife and cut our head off."

"Do you think he means it?" I wonder aloud.

Mrs. Stewart responds sincerely. "Yes, I think he does."

"Do you think the team realizes that?"

"I don't believe they do. I do not believe they do."

Mr. Stewart interjects. "He's threatened to hurt his momma with scissors, knives, he stabbed Gary with a pencil. She had to dig the lead out of Gary's leg."

"It was over nothing." Mrs. Stewart nods. "There's this problem, right now, that we see. It's getting a bigger house so we can put these guys in separate bedrooms. There's got to be somebody who might be willing to help us. I mean, we've even tried on our own to get a bank loan, just enough money to pay this house off and a couple other bills, and make a down payment on another."

Mr. Stewart jumps in the conversation. "See, we owe less than $4,000 on it, but they won't let us borrow $20,000 on it."

They seem to think I can help them. I wonder if I should tell them that I have no resources to help. I wonder what the team is going to do for them. I wonder if the team knows about their needs.

I try to listen for some activity on the part of the team. "So what's happened since the last team meeting? Has anything happened? Anybody done anything?"

"You mean as far as the team?"

"Yeah."

"Not really."

"We haven't heard from anybody," Mr. Stewart comments.

Mrs. Stewart jumps in. She is in "need" mode again. "The main thing we need, I need to get Kevin's Medicaid switched, but I haven't called yet because he has a meeting with his psychiatrist, and I don't want to mess that up. Cause if we do we won't get his medicine."

I remember that at the team meeting, she was going to change his Medicaid plan so that she could begin going to a new psychiatrist for Kevin. "You're really good about following up and taking care of things you need to take care of," I affirm.

"I have to be. I'm no stranger to hard work. When I was Kevin's age, I used to unload 150-pound feed bags out of my dad's car for our animals. Chicken feed, horse feed, cattle feed."

"Did you grow up on a farm?"

"We had one horse, we had cattle, we had chickens, and we had pigs. So we're used to hard work."

"I would say so," I respond. I try to bring the conversation back to the team. "What do you think the team thinks of you and your family?"

"I hope they like us."

"Do you think they do?"

"I think some of them do. The others don't really know us that well yet. I'll put it like this, this is something my mother taught me. I was raised up to believe whatever your family needs, no matter what it may be, you do whatever you have to, to get it. That's why I say whatever Kevin needs, he's going to get. It doesn't matter what it's going to take."

"Even if it comes down to a residential treatment program," Mr. Stewart adds.

"Exactly," Mrs. Stewart agrees. "He won't like that, but it's what's best for Kevin that's important." I'm surprised at the suggestion. I don't think that the team is discussing that possibility, and compared to other families I've studied, this child doesn't seem to have that level of need. However, I can also imagine how hard it must be to have a child at home you're afraid of.

"What bothers us the most, is him hurting himself or others."

"Of course."

Mrs. Stewart continues. "'Cause see, I can deal with him hurting me. I'll be truthful." She nods toward her husband. "He's the only man who has never in my whole life abused me. Ever. But, when Kevin gets mad, he'll bang his head against the wall, and he's hurting himself. We don't know how to get him to stop. Physically restraining him only works for so long."

"That sounds incredibly frustrating," I comment.

"It is," Mr. Stewart responds.

"He just goes too far. There are many times when I've had to physically sit on Kevin to make him settle down." Mrs. Stewart says.

Mr. Stewart adds to the story. "Sending him to his room for punishment is no good 'cause he just tears up the place. Spanking him don't seem to do any good."

Mrs. Stewart interjects, "So the only thing I know to do is to physically use my own body to restrain him. I wind up getting hurt in the process."

"If you spank him, he'll turn around and laugh at you," Mr. Stewart adds.

I don't know how to respond so I try again to move the discussion to the team. "Do you think your team listens to you?"

"Except for the incidents of violence at home, yes," Mrs. Stewart responds.

"Does your team make you feel important, do you think?" I ask.

She shrugs. "The first meeting we had, they wanted to hear everything we could tell them, and they listened to us. But here lately, he's gotten violent, and it's escalating, and I'm seriously afraid that Kevin's going to hurt himself or his dad or Karla or Gary. 'Cause me, I can live with it. I've been through abuse, so I can take it a lot better than they can. I shouldn't have to take it, but when it comes right down to it, I can stand it a lot better than they can."

"Do you think your team makes you feel like there's something wrong with you or your family?" I wonder.

"In the meetings, they talk like we're one of them. They don't talk down to us like most people do," Mrs. Stewart says.

"Do they make you feel like they care about your family?" I ask.

They nod. "Like Nancy did the home improvement stuff. 'Cause she put herself out on a limb to start with to get us that check. Because they didn't even have the family budget when she did that. She got us bus passes."

"Do you think your team respects your family?" I ask.

"Yes, I do. I really do," Mrs. Stewart answers with a nod of her head for emphasis. "When we go to the meetings, they welcome us, they ask us how we're doing, would we like anything to drink, you know, that kind of stuff. Is there anything we might need for the kids? The only thing I can think is a bigger house. They must have got contacts that we don't. There has to be somebody that could help us get a larger house. I've been looking in house magazines, and I've seen three- or four-bedroom houses for $59,900 on more than an acre of property. I know what to look for."

"We saw one recently that has five bedrooms," Mr. Stewart adds. "The guy wants $56,000 for it, but he don't want to work with us. That's cash."

"We can't do that," Mrs. Stewart says.

Mr. Stewart continues. "The yard ain't very big, but the house is much bigger."

"We could get by with a yard the same size as this if the house was bigger," Mrs. Stewart explains. "Each of the boys could have their own room, and I could have another room where I could put out my sewing and my yarn and get all that stuff out of their room." She points to a pile in the corner of the room. "See, over there is my sewing stuff. My sewing machine sits right over there because I have no place to put it."

"If we had somebody who would work with us," Mr. Stewart adds. "We need money for a down payment, if we sell it while we're living in it."

"Do you think the team is flexible enough about your needs?" I ask.

"I think they are," Mr. Stewart responds. "Like I said, the one thing we really need to address is Kevin's violence. That's the one thing that's not being addressed as it should be."

"See," Mrs. Stewart adds. "I've been having to carry all the weight, because being sole caretaker, I monitor his medicine, Kevin's, my own. I take Karla and Gary to the bus stop every morning, and I get them every afternoon. I cook, I clean, I do all the laundry. If it's raining, he has to go and get them in the van, but other than that, I do it all."

I notice that we've been talking for almost two hours. I move to close the interview. "Is there anything else that you want to say, that you haven't already talked about before I let you go?"

Mrs. Stewart sits forward. "The only thing that I really want to stress is maybe getting help to get a larger house, and Kevin's violence. Right now those are the two main issues."

Mr. Stewart interjects. "There is a more pressing issue; we've got to get this place straightened up because the city code people are coming down on us. They say the place has got to be painted."

"Which I'm doing as I can," Mrs. Stewart adds.

"Is Nancy helping you with that?" I ask.

She shakes her head. "They was supposed to find some people to pitch in and help one weekend, but she hasn't found anybody. I've got the paint. We just need extra hands is all we need."

Mr. Stewart adds, "We got the yard cleaned up. I've been working on the shed a little bit every day trying to extend it so I can take that stuff out there under that car and put it in the shed, 'cause the city said something about it."

As I walk toward my car, I wonder what my butt looks like from the couch. I'm sure I smell like smoke. When I left the house this morning, I felt clean. Very clean. Now I feel dirty. I feel like I have a layer of dirt on me. At least I don't see any more bugs. Hopefully there's none in my purse. I feel itchy. My teeth feel icky. My hair feels icky. I smell icky. Rolling down the window, I hope I can air myself out on the way back to my office.

My thoughts wander as I drive. These people are helpless. No, actually, they're quite self-sufficient. At least, they perform self-sufficiency very well. Are they trying to construct service-worthiness (Marvasti, 2002)? What they are, is hopeless. I'm sitting here trying to figure out if I could get some friends from school or church to come help them clean the place up, and I wonder if it's even doable. I mean, it would be such a huge job, and I just have this really funny feeling that we could kill ourselves to clean the place up, and a week later it would look the same. They remind me of Pigpen from *Peanuts*, who has a cloud of dust and bad luck and troubles just kind of following him around. Maybe trouble is what's being constructed. I don't know. Very interesting and very sad, but my point right now is that I feel very dirty and just very nasty after leaving, and I really wonder what my butt looks like.

Maybe what's going on is a construction of a culture of violence. Or maybe some sort of culture of poverty perhaps. I don't know, and I don't see that the team's doing anything to pull them out of it. I don't think the team at the moment is doing much of anything. I think that they're reinforcing what these people already have, kind of an 'us versus them.' The team's over there, kind of above them, helping them.

But, they are helping them. They're listening to them, but nothing much seems to be happening. I don't know. I'm not sure if this was a good team to study. I just don't think at the moment there's much to study. It will be interesting to see what happens when I talk to the other team members.

What a pitiful house. It's sad. Even if it were cleaned up, it wouldn't be a nice house. It's old, it's falling apart. It should be torn down. It's dirty. It's cluttered. But Mrs. Stewart is right. She's got three kids in one room, and they don't have proper furniture. They don't have places to put things. There's no hope of having places to put things.

It strikes me that years of despair, hopelessness, disenfranchisement, and marginalization cling to everyone who crosses their threshold, cling to them, and to everything in their dark, dusty, cluttered home.

Turning into my golf course subdivision, I think about the challenge to see the family as unique, worthwhile individuals separate from their mental, emotional, cognitive, behavioral, social, and financial problems. That's why a systemic and strengths-orientation is so important. When I realized how small their house was and the implications of having no closets, that made me rethink my judgment of how cluttered their house and yard are. When I saw Mrs. Stewart's crafts, I was able to see her as a holistic person with interests, skills, and talents that, frankly, were not too dissimilar to mine. When I heard about their violence but remembered incidents of violence in my home growing up, I realized in some ways that maybe we're not so different after all. Yet, in the end, when I focused on our differences—the gap between what she has and what I have—it was hard to get past the oppressive heaviness of hopelessness and discouragement.

CHAPTER 3

Abandon All Hope: Challenging Hopelessness

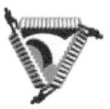

Challenging Deficits

Eating lunch with my colleague Ellen, I tell her about my research. "I'm really having to challenge myself to be strengths-based! They're moving so slowly in helping the family! I'm just having difficulty seeing anything but deficits and problems with the family. And the team. They're just not doing much for the family. There's nothing going on. I hope I have something to write about!"

"You know," Ellen says kindly, "Like me, you are a real problem-fixer. How does that affect the way you're seeing the team?"

I take a bite of lettuce and think. How does that get in the way of my equalizing power in my relationship with the team? I wonder.

On the way home, I'm thinking about how the team doesn't seem to be doing much to help the family, and I wonder why. Do they think the situation is hopeless? Do they think the Stewarts should be doing more to help themselves? I think of the guys with the signs on the side of the road. It occurs to me that, yeah, while it's true that these people could be holding down paying jobs, they clearly don't have the same choices or resources in life that I do. People with the same opportunities as I do not stand on the side of the road for hours on end holding up a sign, waiting for an occasional person to throw change at them.

Communicating Hope: An Ethnography of a Children's Mental Health Care Team by Christine S. Davis, 47–63 © 2013 Left Coast Press, Inc. All rights reserved.

A week later, I park my car on the street outside Washington High and go into the office. The lady there knows me now, and greets me warmly.

"Hi," I say. "I'm here to sit in on Mr. Camelini's class. He said to come on out to his trailer."

"Sure, honey," she responds. "Let me make sure he's there." She picks up her intercom. "Mr. Camelini, Mr. Camelini. You have a visitor."

I can hear his response over the speaker, but I can't make out what he says over the static. It's short, so I assume he's saying "okay."

"Go on out, honey. They're coming back from playing basketball," she says with a smile as she chews what I assume is gum.

I hesitate. "I don't know which is his trailer."

"Third one on the left, across the field."

As I cross the field, I see Mr. Camelini and Kevin in the distance. Kevin sees me and runs up to greet me. For a moment I think he's going to hug me, but he stops before he does.

"Hi, Kevin!" I say. I wonder if he greets everyone this way, or if he remembers me. I can't imagine how he would. I met him only the one time, at the first team meeting, and he was pretty emotionally distraught the whole time. "I'm Mrs. Davis. I'm working with the people who are helping your family."

"I know who you are," he answers, almost with impatience.

I walk up the stairs to the trailer, with Kevin accompanying me closely. Mr. Camelini offers me a chair in the front of the room, and Kevin sits next to me.

"Kevin, you have to return to your seat!" Mr. Camelini insists, but Kevin shakes his head and refuses to budge. I move to a desk on the student side of the room, hoping that Kevin will follow, but he instead moves to the chair I vacate.

As I wait for Warren to arrive and the rest of the students to return to the room, I look around. Because it's a portable and a special-needs classroom, I had expected it to look different from a "normal" classroom. However, it has lots of "classroom" symbols around. A chalkboard at the front of the room. An alphabet tacked across the board. There's a calendar with the days crossed off. I wonder if that's for the benefit of the students or the teacher. A small television is mounted on the wall, next to a large black-and-white clock and a small flag. The student desks are large, with attached plastic seats. There's a metal desk in the front of the room and a small kitchen in the back. Mr. Camelini is grading papers. I watch him for a moment. An older grandfatherly type man, with white hair and a white mustache, he seems very gentle-mannered and quiet-spoken.

Mr. Camelini had told me that there are nine kids in the class; today three boys file in from the field. I understand from conversation that one is suspended and one is helping play Santa for a special program. I don't know where the rest are.

Warren arrives and, despite the fact that he knew I was coming, takes a minute to register who I am. He's a tall, imposing man. He takes off his leather coat and hat with the style of a man who's sure of himself. He remembers the names of all of the kids. I think it's his third or fourth time he's visited Mr. Camelini's class.

He writes two headings on the board: "Role Models" and "Your Personal Style."

"A role model is someone you want to emulate, be like," he explains to the kids. He seems to have their rapt attention. He used to be a professional athlete, and both his physical and personal presence can capture a room. "A role model could be a community leader. Who's your role model, Cedric?"

"My mom and dad," Cedric answers.

Warren nods. "Good, good," he affirms.

He moves to the second column on the board. "Your own personal style." He turns to one of the boys. "Why were you suspended? Why were you fighting? You felt you had to stand up to them. Let them know you're the man." The kid nods. "Got you suspended. Is there a better way to handle it?" The kids are all watching him intently, including Kevin who's still at the front of the room sitting next to the board.

One kid ventures a guess. "You can tell."

"You can tell, but then you're a snitch," Warren responds. "Is there another way?"

"You can walk away."

Warren repeats, "you can walk away." He pauses to let that sink in. He turns to another boy. "He'll look like a punk. What can he do?"

"Talk to him?" another kid ventures.

"What kind of conversation can you have?" Warren asks.

"Talking don't work!"

"In most places it should work but it doesn't," Warren responds. "Why?" He turns this into a teachable moment and writes on the board. He continues talking: "Low self-esteem and peer pressure. You're dealing with yourself. Everybody has peer pressure. It's all in how you think. With high self-esteem, you can talk somebody out of fighting. You can control other people. Now the new kid on the block," I know he's talking about Kevin, but I'm not sure the other kids do. "The new kid on the block has low self-esteem. You can pick him up and help him have high self-esteem, and he won't have to fight."

He explains how responses escalate, and I note that this is the best explanation of the theory of "degenerating spirals" I have ever heard. He turns to the boy in the front row. "Tell me what you understand."

The boy explains the concept better than any undergraduate student in my Interpersonal Communication class could. "If I get mad at him, then he gets mad at me, then I fight, and he fights back, then I fight more, and he fights more."

Warren continues. "You got to learn how to stop it, how to handle it differently. Walk away. Laugh. Learn how to talk, it's what you say. You can't talk back negative. You have to talk back positive."

He calls a boy up to the front of the room. "You want to fight me? Why you want to fight me?" He acts as if he's going to fight, then he walks away from him. "I had to step back," he explains. "On the streets you have to be able to survive." He tells a story of two kids who were fighting and gambling. He says that kids with low self-esteem carry a weapon. "High self-esteem has respect for others' property and space."

"You shouldn't let other people's style take your style away," Warren explains. "Kevin, whose style do you like?" he asks.

"Ernest," Kevin answers.

"Ernest, what do you like about Kevin's style?"

Ernest thinks for a minute. He is a big kid, at least three times Kevin's size, tough looking. He smiles. "What I like about Kevin," he says with a swagger, "is that he don't care how big you is, he won't back down!" I remember that it is this quality that has gotten Kevin in serious trouble many times.

A boy named Corey speaks up. "Kevin can spell and read anything. He can read medical journals!"

"Yeah," Warren says. "Kevin has heart! Everybody has some style that everybody likes."

I find out that Warren is doing these lessons weekly for Mr. Camelini's class. I wonder how they're making a difference.

The Dollar

That Sunday, our minister at church gives us each a one-dollar bill with an assignment—find a way to use this dollar to multiply it for God's service. I think a lot about what to do with it. I think about asking people at school or work to give matching donations, but I rule that out—it's too pushy. Finally, I decide to put it in my car and give to the next guy begging on the side of the road. It doesn't seem like very much, so I go through my wallet and take out more one-dollar bills. I put the stack of bills in the center console of my car, where I can reach it easily. I don't have to wait long for my chance to use it.

Does the Family Have Dreams?

My meeting with Jane, the SED specialist from Washington High, is the following Tuesday. She's a no-nonsense woman, friendly and casual. She's dressed in a denim jumper and tennis shoes. I remember she was in tennis shoes at the team meeting as well. I cannot imagine having her job, dealing with problem teenagers all day long. I ask her about it. "How did you come to do this job?"

"I have a degree in Social Work, EH, and Educational Leadership. It was a fluke," she says. "They put me in a high school, and I kind of liked it. I've been doing it for 20 years."

"What do you like about it?" I ask.

She smiles. "It's always different. You never know."

"How did you get involved with this team?" I wonder.

"Kevin was sent to us with behavior problems left, right, and center," she explains. "They beat him down, so they sent him to us. If he misbehaves, they come to me. But lately there really hasn't been anything. I was out for a week, and there was the bus problem. He threw something and hit the bus aide, and they took him off the bus for two days, and he was suspended."

"How do you interact with Nancy?" I ask.

Jane shrugs. "I normally don't really interact with her at all, unless she calls me with something she needs, or if she's setting up a meeting. I've worked with her on occasion with other kids, so that's how I know her."

"How do you typically interact with the other members of the team?" I ask. "The other people who are helping Kevin?"

She responds, "I know Warren is going to Mr. Camelini's class, but I haven't even seen him; I just know he's coming. I see Mr. Camelini if there's a problem or if Kevin's doing A-OK, he'll come to tell me that, or Kevin comes to me and tells me everything is fine. Peggy and I just roll along dealing with other kids."

I notice how casual and matter-of-fact she is about her job. As we're sitting in the interview, sounds of fighting can be heard outside her door. Washington is without a principal, so she is playing both roles. Today, she is hiding out with me in her office doing this interview. She's managing to ignore the chaos outside her door.

I move on to my next question. "So of all the team members, you and Peggy probably communicate the most. What do you guys talk about?"

"Either a student having a behavior problem, or a home problem, or this child has this going on, or this change. Medication issues, school issues, home issues."

"When you're talking about this family, what kinds of things do you talk about?" I wonder.

"Basically his cleaning," Jane says. "How Peggy gave him a lot of clothes and she hasn't seen them on him. Shoes, clothing, he comes to school dirty. She told me what the house looked like, but I'd already heard it from the bus driver. She said she'd never seen anything like it before."

"What do you think about that?" I ask. "I've interviewed the family, and I've been to their house—what's the deal? I mean, this is not my area of expertise."

Jane leans forward. "Honestly, and I am not a psychologist, but a lot of times when you have people who are poor, they hold on to everything. They're doing the best they can with what they have, which isn't a lot. I mean, if a parent asks for help, and she wants a bathtub, what does that tell you?"

I'm a little surprised and impressed with her level of compassion. I think of other teams I've observed in which school staff blame the parents for their poverty, and I don't hear that in her voice.

"What do you think the team is trying to do for them?" I wonder.

"Nancy said they're going to try to get the behavioral specialist in their home. I think that's wonderful. To get someone who's objective in there and show them this is not the way to live. You can see how Mrs. Stewart honestly doesn't see anything wrong with the way they're living, which is why I think the problems go back to Mom and Dad. He's not EMH— they read on a second-grade level, and Kevin's not that low-functioning. I think they need to work with Mom first, because of the house. Kevin had flea bites all over him." She sits back in her chair, then repeats: "She's doing the best she can with what they have."

"As a member of the team, what are your goals for them?" I ask. "What do you want for the family?"

"I don't know if they can see anything else, to be honest. If they can get somebody in there to help show Mom the way, that would help a lot. But Mom has her own problems that aren't touched."

"What about for Kevin?" I ask.

"I hear a lot of things, but I don't know what's going on. I don't want to call Mom, 'cause it's not really my business. My business is with Kevin at school. He's definitely babied. But her letting him attack her? No. You have to set your boundaries. She hasn't put her boundaries down. He'll throw tantrums. Don't allow tantrums, you know?"

I wonder if it's that easy. Kids do a lot of things that parents don't want to allow them to do. "Could you describe the team meeting from your point of view?"

Jane responds, "When we go there, I'm not informed. I'd like to know what is going on, so when we sit down, maybe the team meetings are more than putting together all the information."

I think for a second. "So, that might be one purpose of the team meeting, perhaps sharing information. Are there any other purposes or functions of these team meetings?"

Jane shakes her head. "I've never sat in a meeting like that before. Just to get on the same page, to see if there's anything else we can think of. To put together everyone's view to see what the total picture is."

"Do you think you're making a difference, getting together and talking?" I wonder.

"Honestly, I have no idea," Jane says with a wave of her hand. "But he's improving. I don't know if that's because something is going on at home, or if it's for real. Or, does he not want to lose his points that he's made? 'Cause he's happy with that. He's learned that he's moving up, and the points can be used in the school store, and he's been there a few times now."

I shift gears. "Let me ask you about a few observations I have and then see your take on them. Mrs. Stewart seems to be a very emotional person. I wonder if that rubs off on him."

She nods. "How could it not? This family orientation and emotions, it runs in families. Families that are loud and hugging and kissing and very overzealous, the child is the same way. She's over-the-top, and he's over-the-top. That's a learned behavior. There may be something there that we don't know about."

"Yeah," I say. "Absolutely. She's very upset and emotional. She clearly cares a lot. She's clearly engaged in helping him."

"It may not be in her capacity to change things, at this point," Jane suggests.

"What does that do for you guys, working with her?" I ask.

"He's getting better. I think he can be maintained," Jane says.

"So really what I hear you saying, and I've been observing this, too, is you can help him without helping the whole family, although it would be better if you could work with the whole family," I summarize.

"It would be better if we could help all our families," Jane says with a nod of her head. "But we can't. But we can help the kid. That's what we're supposed to do."

"It's interesting—you say you can't help the child without helping the whole family, yet that seems to be what the team is doing, helping the whole family," I note. "I wonder if helping him at school is also helping their family situation."

"We have a lot of parents, when a kid improves at school, they tell us that things improve in the home. They're not as combative, or yelling back or doing this—they actually come home and say 'I like school.' He's not fighting with his brothers and sisters. He talks to me now, he doesn't yell at me. We have a lot of kids for whom here's where we see success. Not at home. Obviously he didn't get here for being successful."

"What is it like to be involved with a child and family team? What's the experience like?" I ask.

"When you sit down, you get the whole picture. Because I tell teachers—have you looked at this kid? Have you actually seen what the kid's gone through? No? You need to."

I make a mental note of her emphasis on focusing on the entire system—the family, the environment, the context.

"How do you keep from feeling hopeless about their situations?" I wonder.

Jane shakes her head. "I don't ever think that, so I can't tell you how I stay out of it, 'cause I don't think that way."

"How do you think?" I ask.

"I think, we haven't gotten there yet," Jane says. "We might not get there on all of them, but we get there on some."

Focusing on future possibilities constructs hope.

"What do you think it's like for the parents and the families, to be on this team?" I ask.

"She probably feels anxiety. Kevin probably likes it 'cause he likes getting the attention. He likes any kind of attention."

Hmmm, I think. "What do you think this team thinks of this family?"

She clarifies. "What do I think?"

"Yeah. What do you think?"

"They have a long way to go," she says. "How did they get this far without help? How come all along he wasn't referred to something? All along, this is not an average family. I don't understand how it's gotten this far."

I move on to my next question. "Do you think this team treats this family as if they are an equal member of the team, that they have equal voice, equal power?"

"They still sit and listen. They don't cut Mom off. She talks until she's done. Isn't that how you empower someone, by listening to them?"

Is it? I ask, "Do you think the team makes the family feel like they have dreams?"

Jane is frank. "That the family has dreams? I don't know if they have dreams at all, to be honest. I'll bet they've never been to Disney World. Do they go to movies? Do they go to the pool? Do they go to the beach? 'Cause they don't do family things. Like she wants to have a car—they can't afford that. If someone would just for once take them out into a different world and let them see how it is. 'Cause they beat you down and you never come out. They know nothing else."

Is a family without dreams, a family without hope? I wonder. "Do they have strengths?" I ask.

"They're together as a family. A mother *and* a father. They have a house. She cooks for them. They take care of each other."

"I wonder if she sees that as strengths," I say.

"Probably not. Because she has no clue what's out there," Jane says.

"Do you think the family feels the team has compassion for them?" I ask.

"I'm not really sure if they know that emotion at all. I feel bad for them, but I don't know if they think of compassion. I think they feel lost and they don't know what to do. Here's Kevin who's definitely a different character, and she's trying her best, and she hasn't succeeded. Their problems are in everyday living, not hopes and dreams and where are we going on vacation. That's not even in their vocabulary. That's not in their realm of anything they think about, I'm sure."

"Do you think the team affects that at all, the way they see themselves, the way they feel?" I wonder.

"Probably not. But the team could probably help them by just going in and helping. You can talk till you're blue. But actually going in there. Get volunteers to help clean out their house. Show her that there's compassion out there in the world to help them, not just tell them. Show them," Jane says, emphasizing the last sentence.

"Do you think the team respects the Stewarts?" I ask.

"Respects them? Accepts them the way they are. I just accept them the way they are. This is the situation. Mom's not drinking, smoking, doing drugs, she's not running around. She's trying to hold them together. You have to respect them for that."

"Is it hard not to be judgmental with this family?" I wonder. "It would be real easy, I think, to look down on this family. It seems like it would be easy to judge them or to think badly of them." I think of many other team meetings I've attended in which people seem to blame the family for their problems.

"I don't blame them, because I don't think they know any better. This situation—yes, they created it, but that's all they know. How can you blame them? You can't blame them for being uneducated in the world. Who knows what her life was? She's doing the best she can. She's not lying on her butt, not taking care of her kids, sitting in the projects, blaming everyone else for her problems. She's not blaming anyone for her problems. I don't blame them."

"You sound very compassionate toward her," I notice.

"What can I do? What is, is. You can't change what is. You can change what will be. She listens. They've probably had nothing but despair. By talking to her, you can see it. Despair. But she probably doesn't know it's despair, if that's how you live. How do you know? Do they ever go to McDonald's, on a family outing? What we take for granted—hop in the car, go to the mall, have Chick-fil-A. They don't do that. You know they don't do that. They probably walk to the corner store, to go for groceries."

"What about Kevin? What's his future?" I ask.

"Kevin will be okay. He'll always be off-keel of what the average and normal human being is, because his environment, that's all he knows. He hasn't seen the opportunities. He has no clue."

"So is part of helping them about breaking the cycle?" I respond.

"Mm-hm," Jane affirms.

I wonder. "Do you think you guys can do that? Break the cycle?"

"I think he needs therapy. They've got this therapist coming into the house. If you can change the family dynamics, that will help Kevin."

"What else would you like to tell me about this team, your work, or this family, that I haven't asked you about?" I ask.

"They need people in there to help them. It would be nice if they just went somewhere. A trip to the mall, to the beach. Have they ever been to the beach? Have they ever seen the water? Take them to the beach. Take them to Busch Gardens. Let them have fun and forget their worries for a day."

"Yeah!" I suddenly feel hopeful about this family.

"What does Mom wish for?" Jane asks. "Does she have any hopes and dreams? I don't think she does. But offer; she probably has them somewhere. What did you want for your life? What did you want to do? What changed that? What did you want to do when you grew up? Where do you see yourself in 5 years, 10 years? What do you want to accomplish?"

I leave her office deep in thought. It occurs to me that this is the first time I've been shown the family's strengths.

Things Are Going to Get Harder

At home, I pick up the paper to unwind from my day. On the front page of the Metro section, I see a headline: "Child welfare won't give parents details of baby's death, story on page 4." I turn to page 4 and read. The parents of a 3-month-old boy got into a fight at their apartment, and the sheriff was called. Child welfare removed the boy from their home, and the state was later awarded custody of him. Three weeks later, the baby was found dead at his foster home; no one knows why, and the parents can't get any details. I think how awful and helpless they must feel.

The next morning, Nancy and I pull into her parking lot at the same time. She parks her Lexus and greets me warmly. Nancy is a woman with style, sleek and sophisticated. Today she's wearing what appears to be a silk teal-colored pants suit that sets off her blonde hair perfectly. The Center for Children and Families' office is a portable trailer on the grounds of an elementary school. We navigate around a line of small children as Nancy fishes in her purse for the door keys. We find an empty office and chat as I pull out my tape recorder for our interview. Nancy watches me set up the microphone as I move papers out of my way from the corner of the desk.

I start with a background question as I settle into the cushion of the desk chair. "Tell me about your background, what you did before you were with The Center for Children and Families."

"I was a therapist," she responds. "I was in private practice, and I was really satisfied. I got a call about this particular project, looking at certain kinds of approaches to a systems management kind of coordination, which I thought really needed a lot of work and attention, but I wasn't sure it needed to be from me. It's been an adjustment—the family being a partner at the table, not coming to take from your expert knowledge, so it's a different role."

"Tell me about that," I ask.

Nancy shifts in her chair. "As a therapist, my role was to go to the DSM-IV and give somebody a diagnosis. We operated under a medical model. You might remember to focus on strengths, but you're still following a medical model."

"What is it like now?" I'm fascinated by how well this fits into my thesis.

"My role as a team leader, I'm very comfortable with that. I've had to change my thinking though, that you can offer information and suggestions, but you have to realize whether they want to use it is their decision."

Interesting. "How would your interaction be different from when you were a therapist?"

"As a therapist, I'd go into their problems more deeply. In the role I'm in now, I know what the issues are, but there are more boundaries. I'm not their therapist. Now, I really want them to be more a partner at the table." She pauses for a minute and begins again, this time with a teaching tone of voice. "When you're in the role of a therapist, you are by nature putting yourself in the role of kind of an expert, and it's not a role of equality. The role of a team leader, people have a lot of needs, but you have to keep the boundaries in place."

Boundaries seem to be a big issue with this team in a lot of ways, I think. "Let's talk about this family in particular. Tell me about your experiences with them."

"If I was their therapist, instead of reminding the family that they need to have a neurological workup done with Kevin, instead of suggesting that they do more follow-up on that, I would be pushing it very hard," Nancy says. "Because I think that he really has some significant possible organic issues that might show up in a more thorough neurological workup. I would ask that they be looking at family education and therapy. The medical center has given them very little mental health treatment, and we haven't been able to get the mental health people to the table in the team either, so I think he's getting sort of minimum involvement, and he needs maximum. I really think he needs a lot more medical assessment, and to get the parents involved in some parenting lessons."

"So how do you feel about the fact that you can't do that?" I ask.

Nancy shakes her head. "It's sometimes frustrating. I give people more autonomy in their decision making than I might have before. But even as a therapist, you cannot—well, you can force them to do something, but I haven't found it to be a real success, forcing people to do something they're not ready to do."

I imagine not. "Yet," I say, "helping patients to take an active role in their own care is essential to empowering them" (Stylianos & Kehyayan, 2012).

"Right," Nancy says. "That's my job to help educate them, advocate for them. Not force them. You can't force someone to be empowered."

I nod. "Tell me about this family."

"This family has some pretty basic economic and social needs," Nancy responds. "It's challenging, because there are chronic health issues, chronic financial issues. I would say kind of daily functioning, daily living kinds of things. There are so many needs there that sometimes the mental health component gets neglected, because the basic needs are being attended to. It's often a crisis," she adds.

"How does this team operate with the family?" I wonder.

She pauses for a minute before answering. "It's an educational process, because at school, they have more than the usual challenges with Kevin. So their initial focus was, how do we get him to settle down and do some academic work? My experience tells me that we have not yet identified exactly what is wrong with Kevin, and exactly the best way to help him. His teacher is a very dedicated person. But he doesn't know what to do, because everything he's used with other kids successfully doesn't necessarily work with Kevin."

I see this in my mind's eye. "What's the best interaction this team has?"

"They're always willing to meet. I can tell they're very interested in Kevin and about making things work. Also, I think there have been incidences with him when he first came to that school, that if not for this team, he would have been suspended already. There was a bus incident that frankly was a big safety issue, and I'm surprised that he wasn't suspended no matter what the school wanted to do. There have been several times that I think the frustration level at the school has been so high that they would have just given themselves a rest by suspending him, but they haven't. They've continued to work with him. I just think they would like some help in knowing how."

"You know," I say, "this makes me think of the ongoing challenges of empathizing with clients, children, and families without marginalizing them. I've noticed how you each use humanizing language to see this family as whole people, beyond their problems, and to understand the situation from their point of view. I think you team members are amazingly able to put yourselves in the place of the family. I also think of what a challenge it is to move the family from crisis mode to empowerment mode. It seems very difficult to build a family's resources, capabilities, and hopes while simultaneously fixing urgent problems. I notice you begin working on the crises before moving to resource-building, but what if a family never moves out of crisis mode?"

Nancy looks thoughtful. "Well, dealing with crisis and moving the family into the future, giving them something to hope for both in the present and the future, must sometimes be done at the same time. Crisis should not prohibit empowerment."

I nod. "What would you say is the worst interaction the team has had?" I wonder.

"In the very beginning, when the people were trying to form as a team, and they didn't know much about us, and I could see them asking, 'Who's going to help us do something about this kid? Is it the family? Is it these people from the Center for Children and Families? Who is it?' It really wasn't a team. Since then, it's become more of a team."

I'm surprised at her last comment and decide to challenge her on it. "From what I'm observing, they still don't seem to be a team. There wasn't much interaction with the family at the team meetings, I thought. Except for school people talking to school people, there doesn't appear to be a lot of conversation as a team."

"There's not much as I'd like to see," she admits. "At least they're starting to think of themselves, at least in some sense, as a team."

I'm especially interested in this observation. "What makes you think that?"

She taps the table as she talks. "They talk to one another about Kevin. In the last team meeting, if you remember, they were talking about coming to a consensus about how they would handle certain behaviors of Kevin's." She's right; they did do that. "I do think you're right that there's not much team interaction with the parents. Maybe that's the nature of working with the school—there's no principal at that school, and that school is just brimming with too many kids. They don't have any place to meet. They get discouraged dealing with one crisis after another."

I hesitate for a second before mentioning my next observation. "If I were on that team, I would not be that eager to be going out to their house and spending a lot of time with them. It's really dirty. I hope I'm not being too unkind."

"That's reality," she agrees. "To be very blunt about it, it's not pleasant to go to that home. There's no place that you feel comfortable sitting down. Everything in the house is very dark. The house is brimming to the rafters with all kinds of stuff. Both the parents smoke continually, and I can hardly breathe. The house is so dirty that there has been actual conversation at our staff meeting about where you draw the line. You heard at that one meeting that Kevin didn't come to school clean. It's not that they don't want to do anything about it. They clearly don't even realize it. Their standard of living is so different. The city has cited them about the mess in their yard, and they became very incensed about it. They don't recognize it."

"Do you think it's their culture or a symptom of problems?" This is something I've been wondering all along.

"I think it's both. Some cultural, but I think it's deeper than just cultural. I think it's symptomatic. The household is very disorganized, which is interesting, because the mother is very organized about making and keeping appointments. She doesn't lose things."

"I wonder if that's related to Kevin's problems?" Am I doing what I've accused team members of, wrongly blaming the parents for the kids' problems?

Nancy shrugs. "You can't get a good breath of air in there, and I wonder if Kevin has any personal space. I've never been there when the TV isn't on. I've never gone there when the parents are not watching TV. So I wonder, where do the kids read? Where do they do their homework? Where do they just go? The basic stuff, your own space, cleanliness, organization, Kevin doesn't have that."

"She's one of the most self-sufficient people I think I've ever met," I say. "Even her husband, who's got all these disabilities, it's incredible how much they do for themselves." I try to turn our discussion toward strengths, because I'm afraid that I moved us into deficit mode with my previous question.

"She certainly does have that appearance, but she doesn't drive," Nancy points out. "She has money in her budget to get her driver's license and take driver's education, and it's been in there for four months."

I nod and move on to my next question. "Tell me about your relationship with the other members of the team." I ask.

Nancy smiles. "I knew Jane prior to Kevin attending there, and she's a person who really does care about the kids. She's been very cooperative, and he hasn't gotten suspended, and he has really pushed the limit at that school. I hadn't known Mr. Camelini before. He doesn't seem to fit in; this is a tough school in a tough neighborhood. He seems to sincerely want to do just the right thing to help Kevin. Warren—one of the most dedicated people I work with—referred Kevin. He really loves kids, especially Kevin. He was so concerned about Kevin, and so desperate for something to help him, and he knew Kevin didn't fit very well into the system. So he was looking for some way that the system could help Kevin. Warren recognizes that Kevin is an outsider at this school. He's around a bunch of tough kids, and Warren's worried about him. Kevin gets around big kids and says something inappropriate to them, like he doesn't understand the consequences of what that can do. Peggy, I've known her before. She's also real good at working with these kids, but she has too many kids to work with. She can't see all very much. You get a lot of frustrated professionals, I think."

"What do you think it's like to be a member of the team?" I am curious as to what her answer will be, as the team leader.

"There are a lot of needs here, and I think it's frustrating that the needs are so overwhelming at times. Everyone says they're willing to do whatever they can, but they're not getting to the bottom of this home situation, and this is a huge challenge. They want to do all that they can to help Kevin. I think that they're kind of wondering what to do. What can I do as a member of the team to counteract what he lives with at home?"

I move to my next question. "Where do you see the team going from here? What's your vision for the team of what you're going to do next?"

"One person I'd like to add to the team would be an educator within the family, to actually help with some organizational skills at the home. I would like to see Kevin have kind of a Big Brother person, which was disrupted when he changed schools. The team has a limited amount of time, and if they did that for every kid in the school they'd be meeting all day long. This team is in conflict with their regular roles."

"Do you think that this team makes this family an equal member of the team?" I wonder.

Nancy shakes her head. "I think they're really respectful of the parents, and I think that they are appropriate in team meetings, but no, I don't. This is a very needy family. It's not that they're separating themselves according to being professionals or trying to stand off, but I think they're really worried about the kind of daily living, functioning of the family."

"Are you saying that if I see ways I can help you, that that makes us not equal?" What an interesting thought.

"Here's an illustration. Before the last team meeting, Jane told me that Kevin's clothes and body were not clean. She was very concerned and even blunt about it, and told me she was going to bring it up in the team meeting. But in that meeting, she didn't say a word about it. It's really hard to address that kind of an issue with a parent, and it's very hard to sit across the table from somebody and say, 'your child is arriving at school in the morning not clean.' Because this is an adult that you're talking to."

"Do you think that the family has equal voice?" I wonder.

"Oh yeah. I have never seen them not listened to at the meeting or not be treated respectfully," Nancy responds with a nod of her head.

"Do you think they have equal power in the meetings?" I ask.

"Yeah. I haven't seen them not get anything that they asked for," she says.

I pause momentarily. Is getting everything you ask for the same thing as having equal power? I wonder to myself. "Does the team communicate in a way that says they have compassion for the family, do you think?" I ask.

"I really do think so," she responds thoughtfully. "They have to take a bus over there, with Mr. Stewart's disability, sometimes on a walker, sometimes on a scooter. I think he's obviously having a really hard time. I think they're compassionate about that, about his physical challenges. I think they're compassionate about Kevin. I don't see anybody on that team that wouldn't want to help Kevin or do right by him, no matter how frustrated they get with him." I think back to my observations and interviews and mentally agree with her.

"So what's next for the team, do you think?" I ask.

Nancy thinks for a minute, then responds quietly. "I think things are going to get harder. I'm past the stage of rapport-building and assessment, and I think there are some real hard issues with this family. They've got three kids that are all going to be getting older, two boys that are in a continual crisis. They've got more health problems than we knew about. I think it's going to get harder, because I think some of the issues we're going to have to talk about, I think they'll be hard things to talk about."

Interesting. I continue. "What's the best you could hope for this family?"

"I think their continual issues are how to survive financially. Mr. Stewart's health is not going to get better. That's going to be more of a challenge. The best we can hope for is to get them some parenting education. What I hope for Kevin is to help him have the most successful kind of day that he can have at school, maybe to give him somebody to spend time with him that would broaden his horizons a bit, give him more exposure to things he would enjoy. I hope we can get to that, to at least help his life be a little more comfortable."

Broaden his horizons. Dream, maybe?

CHAPTER 4

Appearances Are Deceiving: Constructing Turning Points

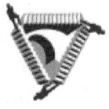

Team Building

The team and I are in Washington's "time-out" room again. I've decided to hold our first team focus group here, to make it easier for everyone at the school to attend. This is easier on the Stewarts also, because they can take a bus directly here. As I explain the meeting process, I unpack the deli sandwiches, cookies, and soft drinks that I brought and put the food on one of the student desks lining the wall. The room is cluttered with desks and books.

"Remember, you've signed consent forms. We're videotaping the meeting today." I point to Alan, who is standing behind my tiny video camera. "Alan is here as my videographer. I think everyone here knows Alan from the Center for Children and Families. He's their Executive Director. Nancy's boss," I add with a smile to Nancy.

He waves to the group as I point. He knows most of the staff from Washington High, and they greet him as old friends.

"Alan is here to run the video camera, and also as a stand-by clinical therapist, just in case there is an emotional crisis, or if anyone in the group needs his help," I continue my explanation. "In case you're worried about your hair today or something like that, I'm the only one who's going to

Communicating Hope: An Ethnography of a Children's Mental Health Care Team by Christine S. Davis, 65–93 © 2013 Left Coast Press, Inc. All rights reserved.

be viewing this tape, and I'm just going to be taking notes on the communication process. So you're okay."

"Then it's going to self-destruct?" Peggy asks.

"It will," I assure them. "You'll all look great on film. Remember, I'm on this tape, too, so I promise that it will be destroyed when I'm done." I add the next line in deference to IRB requirements. "I need to point out the obvious, that you're speaking in a group, and you're speaking in front of your other child and family team members, so just be aware of that."

"In other words, everybody watch your colorful metaphors," Mrs. Stewart adds.

"Whatever you're comfortable saying in front of the others is fine with me," I assure her with a smile. I notice that they're all sitting comfortably around the make-shift conference table, leaning back in their chairs with their arms in an open posture. Several of them are eating the lunch I brought. Smells of pickles and potato chips waft by.

I've struggled with what to talk about in this focus group. I had planned to ask them about their team, but it's occurred to me as I've gone through the interviews and observations that they don't yet seem to me to be a team. Thus, I'm going to ask them what they think a team should be like. "What is important to you for a team to do?" I ask.

Digressions and Crises

Mrs. Stewart answers first.

"Listening. Listening is one of the most important things, 'cause if nobody listens, then nothing's ever going to get done. Kevin's behavior is beginning to get worse, more physically violent." Her voice gets louder. "Yesterday him and Gary started fighting. I got it broke up, and then they came out in the living room and they started all over again. So I did the only thing I knew to do; I spanked them both. After I pulled Kevin off of Gary and spanked him, I moved Kevin aside and when I went to spank Gary, Kevin hits me right in the back with his fist. I'm not even looking at him."

"I wasn't home," Mr. Stewart interjects. "I had to go to my father's house."

"The violence is escalating," Peggy observes.

Mrs. Stewart adds, "I don't want to put Kevin in jail. It could make it worse than what it already is. I don't know what to do." She makes direct eye contact with the team. Her voice is animated.

Mr. Stewart leans forward. "He tells us that he hates us. He tells his mother that she's not his real mother."

"I don't know what to do," Mrs. Stewart repeats.

I think about how I should handle this digression from my focus group topic. They're not on task, but I did want to observe how they communicate and interact in a natural setting. I decide to let them go in this direction for awhile. I wonder if Nancy will jump in and direct them, since this seems to be turning into a therapeutic meeting and she is the team leader.

Mr. Camelini addresses Mrs. Stewart. "Kevin says he doesn't care when he really doesn't know what he's talking about. Kevin doesn't understand what the consequences are."

Mrs. Stewart disagrees. "He knows what the consequences are."

Mr. Camelini argues back. "I don't think he does."

Mrs. Stewart says, "He knows what jail is."

Mr. Camelini concedes that point, somewhat. "He knows what jail is, yeah, but he doesn't have that experience. He knows the word jail, but he doesn't know what jail is."

Mrs. Stewart continues to argue her point. "He sees what they do, because we watch a lot of police programs, so Kevin knows exactly what goes on in jail." Her volume escalates. "Something needs to be done, because I've got to stop this violence. I don't like getting hit, but I'm not letting Kevin hit him." She points to Mr. Stewart. "That I will not do. I don't care what Kevin does to me. Kevin's not going to hit him." She waves her arms above her head for emphasis.

Doing What's Best

Mr. Camelini sits forward. "I thought we agreed in the last meeting that you were going to call the police."

Mrs. Stewart is agitated. Her voice is loud and her arms are waving. "I'm walking a tightrope here between what's best for Kevin and what's best for the whole. I don't want Kevin going to jail if I can absolutely help it. If I can do something to prevent him from having to go, I will." Her hand gestures emphasize her words.

Mr. Camelini faces her. "You do want what's best for him, right?" They make eye contact as they talk back and forth, as if no one else is at the table.

"Yes, I want what's best for Kevin, but I don't want to put him in jail unless we absolutely have to. I don't know what to do. I'm trying to do what's best for everybody, and I'm lost. I'm overwhelmed." She raises her hands in a gesture of futility.

I take a quick glance at my facilitation outline. I mentally toss out several questions that we now won't have time for. I wonder about the significance of the group being unable to move from problem-solving mode to metacommunication (communication about their communication). Maybe it's too soon for them. I've made a conscious effort to be less directive than I normally am when facilitating, because I want the team's natural interaction style to have room to be expressed. I'm finding it fascinating that, in the absence of strong leadership from me, Mrs. Stewart seems to have taken over the leading of the meeting.

"Last week, we said that the things you were trying just aren't working," Nancy says. "None of us want to see Kevin someplace locked up. But, if you try everything else and it gets actually dangerous, I don't know that there's going to be a choice."

Mr. Stewart answers Nancy directly. "It's not that Kevin doesn't know the rules. He knows what to do, and what not to do. He chooses not to."

Mrs. Stewart responds: "He doesn't care about the rules. Anybody's rules. School, home, nothing, he don't care."

Nancy offers a suggestion. "One of the things we talked about last week was trying to get a respite person for Kevin, kind of like a Big Brother person. You said that that had helped him before."

Mrs. Stewart nods. "Yes, it did help Kevin before, and I'd like to get it again if possible."

"We're working on it," Nancy says.

"But the person has to be somebody that Kevin will respect, someone he'll listen to. He doesn't listen to us anymore," Mrs. Stewart emphasizes.

Mr. Stewart adds, "I've got an example. We've got an empty field across the street and a big tree over there. I told Kevin, don't be climbing the tree. We don't own the property. If you fall, get hurt, we're in trouble. So what does he do? He turns right around, climbs the tree. I spanked him, he done it again. He does the same thing over and over, even though we tell him no."

"So what does this team need to do?" I ask, trying to move the conversation back to teams, and regain some control over the meeting.

Mrs. Stewart responds. "We need to find a way to get Kevin back to where he was before he started all this violence."

Warren leans forward to the group. "Did the neurologist test come back yet?"

"There was nothing," Mrs. Stewart says. "Other than a slight swelling of the pituitary glands, that was it. So no neurological signs, they're thinking it's possibly a chemical imbalance."

I ask again, "What can this team do? What do you as a team want to be doing for Kevin?"

Mr. Camelini speaks up. "You know in school, since Christmas break, it's been essentially no problem. During the unstructured time, he still gets in trouble occasionally, and he still tries to walk out of my room. When he gets upset, we let him stay in the time-out room until he calms down. But again, he's improved. According to the point sheet he has, it's been 100s. We've learned how to deal with him, I think. We've had certain limits, parameters, and he's learned what those are, and we function with those."

We are briefly interrupted by an intercom. The words are unintelligible, but no one in the room seems to be distracted by it.

Jane shakes her head. "Last week he was suspended for a couple of days. Did you know what he did to the bus aide? He went after the bus aide in the front office. Twice. I have a question. What happened on Friday when I saw him running all around barefoot? He had some naked little tootsies out there running around." Everyone laughs. "He left his boots somewhere."

Mr. Camelini explains. "There was no P.E. class on Friday. We had basketball, and took the class out, so he had his shoes off. Plus he had his shoes off in the portable."

"But he ran up to the nurse with no shoes on," Jane insists.

"He asked to go to the nurse," Mr. Camelini explains. "We didn't think it was a legitimate reason. So we said no. He went up anyway."

"It was. His foot was bleeding," Mrs. Stewart defends him.

"Probably from running barefoot across the field," Warren adds with a laugh.

"No, this was on the side of his foot," Mrs. Stewart replies.

"He didn't have any socks on," says Mr. Camelini.

Mrs. Stewart adds, "He won't wear socks—that's another thing. I'll give him a clean pair of socks twice a week, because he goes through socks a lot faster than his brother and sister do. He'll wear them to school, but he'll come home without them. I don't know what happens to them." She shrugs her shoulders.

Peggy looks back at Mr. Camelini. "So you took care of the problem without letting him do any more running around."

"He did go to the cafeteria and sat on a bench and cooled off for a while," Mr. Camelini explains.

"That's when I saw him." Peggy says. "Jane and I were in the office talking about another student and that's when we saw him. I was fully expecting him to hit the office door, so that's an improvement, that he went and sat on the bench by the cafeteria, and got things under control."

Mrs. Stewart leans forward. "Why won't he do that at home?"

Nancy addresses the team. "I think that's the key, what you were saying about how the team worked together." She looks at Mr. Camelini. "So you're saying that since Christmas his behavior's been better," then she looks at Peggy, "and you're saying that you saw an improvement."

Peggy responds. "He's not disrupting the whole school anymore."

Nancy turns to Mr. Camelini and Warren. "If that's happening, then maybe the team members at school could share what you think is happening at school that might work at home?"

Boundaries and Limits

Mr. Camelini responds. "We've set limits, and we stick to those. No is no."

Peggy adds, "Schoolwide. Everyone's been on board."

"He's learned that if there's a problem and a kid's picking on him, Mr. Camelini comes right to me, we call everybody into my office and read them all the riot act—keep your hands off of Kevin," Jane tells.

Mr. Camelini adds, "As far as what Warren's doing, one of the students who used to pick on him, he now defends him. So I think he's made some inroads."

Warren says, "The major problems now are coming from the bus, and the bus aide and the bus driver need to have those limits also. They need some kind of structure. On the bus, everyone should get treated the same. With Kevin, if you allow somebody to get away with something, he feels he has the same right, and that really sets him off. When he sees another kid get out of their seat or stand up and yell, he feels he can do the same thing. He's going to be defiant."

Jane argues, "He took a rolled-up newspaper in the aide's face and threatened her with it. He threw things and hit one of the bus aides."

Peggy turns to Mrs. Stewart. "Which is the behavior you've seen."

Warren interjects, looking at Jane. "Something has to be triggering him and making him angry to do that. He don't just get up and do things. Do we have cameras on the bus?" Jane and Peggy shake their heads. "With Kevin, if an adult missed somebody aggravating him, he's going to take matters into his own hands. When he's being reprimanded by the bus driver, he already feels this person is not on his side, so he's going to stand up and go toe-to-toe with them." He makes eye contact around the table. "He's spirited. With Kevin there has to be something that triggers him to be set off. He just don't snap off for no reason."

I think to myself how Warren is taking a systems approach, looking for actions and reactions; context and environment; and ways to alter the environment to create changes in Kevin.

Mrs. Stewart disagrees. "You ought to see him at home. I'll give you an example. Saturday morning we all got up, everybody was fine. Nobody was arguing, nothing. The kids sat down for breakfast. Nobody's bothering anybody. Gary's not saying anything to Kevin. Karla's not saying anything to Kevin. Kevin just hauls off and punches Gary for nothing. Absolutely nothing. Nobody's bothering Kevin, nobody's telling him you can't do this, you can't do that. He just hauls off and punches him."

"What happened when that happened?" Peggy asks.

"Kevin got his rear tore off, but before we got to Kevin, Gary punched him back. So we had to get them both," Mrs. Stewart answers. Her voice is loud and animated. Her hands are gesturing in the air.

Warren nods. "I understand. But there's something that's triggering him to hit."

"I don't know what it could be," Mrs. Stewart says.

"The word 'no' will set him off, in school, everywhere," Jane adds.

Mrs. Stewart nods. "I could be going to set the table. I'll say, 'excuse me Kevin.' He'll move aside, but then he'll hit me. Soon as I've gotten where I'm a little past him, he'll haul off and hit me. All I said was, 'excuse me, Kevin.' It's getting out of hand."

I wonder if this is a good time for me to bring the conversation back to my focus group. I decide to wait a few more minutes. Besides, I don't think I can get a word in right now, anyway.

Peggy enters the conversation. "What do you do when he hits you?"

"I take the stuff to the table and then he gets his butt paddled. He knows that hitting is not right," Mrs. Stewart says.

Jane observes, "But that consequence hasn't worked."

Warren suggests, "Take it to the next level."

Mrs. Stewart argues, "That means the police, but I didn't want to go that route."

"He'll only do 24 hours at the jail. He won't be there long," Warren responds.

Peggy adds, "If he's extremely agitated, he may get emergency commitment instead."

Crazy Is as Crazy Does

Mrs. Stewart's voice is loud and tearful. She runs her hands through her hair in frustration. "But that's what I want to prevent. I don't want Kevin winding up in some loony bin."

"Why?" Peggy asks.

"Because Kevin's not crazy. He's disturbed, but he's not crazy," Mrs. Stewart responds.

"If they can help him . . ." Peggy begins.

"If they can help him, okay," Mrs. Stewart interrupts, "but . . ." She stops, then begins again. "If that's what's going to help him, then so be it, but . . ."

Peggy says, "'Cause what you're doing is not working."

"I know it's not working," Mrs. Stewart says defensively.

"Spanking him is not working," Peggy repeats. "Why do you think he hits you?"

"Because he knows that I'll take it. I will not let—I told Kevin—let him hit him." She points to Mr. Stewart.

"You've set a limit with him," Peggy observes.

"I told him, you want to hit somebody, you hit me. I'm not going to let you hit him. I can take it. I have taken it before." Mrs. Stewart is shouting now.

"No!" Peggy interjects loudly. Everyone around the table nods.

"It's not right, but I'd rather he hit me than him," Mrs. Stewart says, pointing to her husband again.

Jane is clearly concerned. "So it starts with hitting, and you haven't done anything, but what if it starts out with something like this and he stabs you. Are you going to call the police then?"

"Yes, I'm going to call the police!" Mrs. Stewart shouts.

Jane pleads, "Don't let it get this far. If you keep not letting a consequence happen, this will get worse."

Peggy's voice is loud with emphasis. "You've given him permission to hit you. You have said, don't hit him, hit me."

Mrs. Stewart argues. "I said I'd rather you hit me but I would also not want to be hit. He knows that. I've told him, I don't like anybody being hit and I don't want to be hit, but if you're going to hit somebody. . . ." Her voice is drowned out by the group.

Their voices are all getting loud. Jane protests, "No! That's giving him permission to hit you."

All communication—verbal and nonverbal, intentional and unintentional—constructs meaning and thus has consequences, I think.

Mrs. Stewart is fighting tears. "So what am I supposed to do?" She shouts and slams the table. "Fine! Fine! I'm calling the police today. I'm having Kevin taken away permanently." She crosses her arms and turns her back to the table.

Nancy interjects, trying to calm down Mrs. Stewart. "Wait a second. What we need to figure out, from Kevin's perspective, is why he's doing this. He's got some purpose in his mind for that behavior. I'm wondering if it hasn't gotten to the point where Kevin himself hardly knows what it is, because he may have just gotten into a cycle of wanting everybody to be in disarray and upset." She is making eye contact around the table and heads are nodding. "He may have gotten to the point where he just wants to have something going. That in itself may be a purpose for his behavior. Not that he's in the kitchen, or not that he shoved his brother, but just that things are kind of quiet and he wants to start something. It's entertaining to Kevin, maybe, to get everybody in a dither."

Mrs. Stewart argues loudly. "But it's not working, it's not working. It's not getting us upset, it's just getting him corporal punishment."

Nancy nods. "Right. I'm wondering, you tried time-out at school, have you tried it at home? Away in another part of your house."

Mrs. Stewart protests, "There's nowhere to put him. If you put him in his room by himself, he'll tear the room up. He punches the walls. He'll take his clothes, Gary's clothes, throw them all over the place. He'll destroy everything he can get his hands on."

"Make him clean it up," Warren comments.

Mrs. Stewart says, "He won't clean it up."

Warren argues, "He won't come out until it's cleaned up."

"We had him in there all day one day," Mr. Stewart says.

Warren responds, "That's good."

Mr. Stewart continues his story. "But he still didn't clean it up—he punched holes in the walls."

Jane joins the conversation. "Then he should fix those, too."

"He won't do anything." Mrs. Stewart hits the table with her fist. "He don't even want to take his turn doing dishes." She blows her nose.

"What do you think will work?" Peggy directs the question to Mrs. Stewart.

Mrs. Stewart shrugs her shoulders. Her voice is still loud and agitated. "Ask God that question, 'cause I don't have an answer anymore! We've tried corporal punishment mostly. We've tried locking up his cards and stuff like that and it don't make a difference." She rubs her eyes, then tells a story of Kevin's misbehaving on Saturday night. The team listens with intent eye contact and head nodding.

"I can hear your frustration, and I can see how it . . ." Nancy begins to affirm.

Mrs. Stewart interrupts. "Kevin doesn't care about anybody but Kevin. That's it."

"Apparently we're doing something at school that's working, and we cannot do corporal punishment," Mr. Camelini points out.

Express Yourself

Everyone seems to be very upset, and emotions are escalating. I think might be a good time to move the subject back to my focus group. I put on my best 'teacher' voice. "Okay. I want you guys to get up; we're going to do an exercise. You're going to cut out pictures from magazines and build a collage that represents all the experiences of this team."

I'm relieved when they comply. Warren and Mr. Camelini get up and pick up magazines, then return to their chairs. Everyone sits in their seats looking through the magazines.

Mrs. Stewart picks up a pair of scissors and a magazine. "You got a psychology book on nightmares? That would be perfect, because Kevin at home is a nightmare."

"What is this supposed to be about?" Jane asks for clarification.

"It represents this group here," I explain.

"I hope you don't think this group is a nightmare," Peggy mentions to Mrs. Stewart with a smile.

Mrs. Stewart responds, "No. Kevin is the nightmare in the middle, and we're the poor souls that are trying to figure out how to solve it."

I sit back and watch them work, cutting and tearing up pages, flipping through their magazines, intent on their task.

There is little talking. Mrs. Stewart shows her picture to the group. "How about this one?" she asks.

"Put it on!" I encourage.

Mrs. Stewart helps her husband with his magazines, and they talk quietly between themselves. "Look at this," she says. "Doesn't that kind of represent Kevin?"

"Got a picture of heaven in there?"

"Here's the peacefulness that we all wish for. How about that?"

"Cut it out. Put it on."

"How about a picture of Kevin? Right there. Always fishy. Kevin's always up to something like a fish. Perfect picture," Mrs. Stewart suggests.

Mr. Camelini and Warren sit in the corner of the table, going through their magazines. They talk quietly as they go through the pictures. "We use food for rewards," Mr. Camelini explains a picture to Warren.

Mrs. Stewart exclaims to the group, "I found a perfect thing that describes Kevin, an alligator. Kevin knows he's unpredictable. One minute he can be nice and quiet like one of these and then the next it's wham!" Everyone is intent on looking at their magazines, and no one responds to her comment.

"It's time to glue them to the poster board," I instruct the group.

They stand side by side to glue the pictures on the paper. Mrs. Stewart glues the pictures for her husband. She continues to glue while Warren and Mr. Camelini watch and eat. Mrs. Stewart comments, "I'm always trying to help. It's one of my failings." She takes the scissors from

Mr. Stewart and cuts his pictures for him. "That's what we wish he would be," she comments, "a good little tiger rather than an alligator."

When they're done, I pick up the collage and tape it to the wall. I look at the pictures—at a smiling Tony the Tiger in front of a cartoon of a man and woman in ski clothes with the caption "Express Yourself!" Headlines declare "Success," "Skill," "Magic," "Come On In!," "Touch Spots," "Mix & Match," "Smart," "Health Intelligence," and "Good Luck!". A series of pictures of sandwiches is next to a picture of an alligator in a swamp. There's a boat with a tanned, swimsuit clad family in it. A yellow and a red M&M point to a chocolate Easter Bunny. A picture of a shelf of pottery bowls and pitchers, overlapping with a frowning woman holding a rolled up chain in her hand, next to a house with a huge stone fireplace nestled in majestic oak trees. Two men fishing. A group of kids playing basketball and a woman leaning over a young boy. Finally, a cartoon in which a child doing his homework asks his mother, "If two negatives make a positive, how come two wrongs don't make a right?"

I ask the team to describe their efforts. "Tell me about this collage. How does that represent this team?"

"I put a couple things on there," Mr. Camelini begins. "This is a teacher helping the student, and you know the primary reason why they're here is to learn. We try to support them in that learning. The food pictures represent our attempt to create a family attitude within the school with occasional cooking in the portable. We try to create an attitude where they can have some respect for each other. It works."

Mrs. Stewart turns to her husband. "You picked out that one," she says.

Mr. Stewart points to a picture. "This picture shows a father and son who do things together." He points to the headline "Express Yourself!" "We have to express ourselves, in order to make everybody understand what we're doing. We got a lot of intelligence here." He looks around the table.

Mrs. Stewart comments, "Kevin's smart. He just don't want to use his smarts for what it's supposed to be." A chorus of agreement moves around the table.

"He truly is smart," Warren agrees.

Mrs. Stewart says, "I wish he would use it in a proper way instead of in a bad way."

Warren tries to lighten the mood. "I think the President of the United States is a smart man, and he uses it for manipulation."

Mrs. Stewart says with a laugh. "I bet Kevin could beat him hands down."

"Get Kevin in politics," Warren suggests as the group laughs.

Scary thought, I think.

Warren stands up and points to the poster. "Here's mine. It's a basketball that represents Kevin. We're trying to get him to this basket in a safe place. On this team, we've got the supervisors from the school system, there's different types of rules. We're looking for the right thing for this young man so we can get him in this basket and get him in a safe place in his life."

"That's cool," Mr. Camelini responds.

Peggy goes next. "I see this team as being really diverse. I picked out some words such as "Mix and Match" and "Smart." I, too, think we have a lot of intelligence here," she points to Mr. Stewart and smiles. "I picked out all this different pottery, 'cause we're all different, but the picture is also real cluttered, 'cause what we're trying to do is all cluttered up; more like just trying to figure out what to do. Finally, "My Magic," 'cause I really think we're going to need a little bit of magic here."

Mrs. Stewart adds, "A miracle."

Mrs. Stewart points to her pictures. The team looks at the poster as she talks. "I picked out this alligator because it actually describes how Kevin can be. One minute he can be nice and quiet, you don't even know he's there. Then the next minute you got that tail whipped around and you're clobbered. This represents the peace that I think the whole team hopes for. It's a nice peaceful, shady, quiet setting, and what this team represents is the peace that we all want to try to give to Kevin, or to help him achieve." I notice that her voice is quiet and calm.

Jane takes her turn. "I picked the boat because I like the boat. That's the kind of boat we have. We're all in the same boat. We're going to have some tough spots, and we're going to need some skill, but I think we're going to have success at the end."

"I believe these next ones were Nancy's," Mrs. Stewart says.

Nancy stands up and points to her pictures. "This says if two negatives make a positive, how come two wrongs don't make a right? It's a mom and a son talking." She is talking to the whole table, as if she is giving a class lecture. She makes eye contact with each person as she talks. "We're talking about logic. This is like the team, we're trying to figure out things about Kevin. If we could figure out what Kevin wants to have, what the purpose is of his behavior, maybe we could have some more good behavior like we have at school. Maybe we could all come together and figure out some things that Kevin would like to achieve, or some way to work together on figuring out what's in his mind." She returns to her seat.

I notice how even in the immediate midst of frustration and challenges, this team has a vision for themselves. It's an image of different people working together, respectfully listening and brainstorming, bringing different skills, ways of thinking, and experiences together to all work toward the same goal—moving Kevin forward, to a safe place in his life. Their imagery moves them beyond frustrations and confusion, past difficulties and challenges, to a vision of success. And hope. They're using their vision to draw their team together and I'm noticing how it becomes a powerful force for change within their system.

The Future Is Now

No one else volunteers to discuss the poster, so I move to my next set of questions. "I'm going to give you some beginnings of sentences and get you to complete the sentences, okay? To me, child and family teams . . ."

"Should work together," Mrs. Stewart and Mr. Camelini say in unison.

"What I like about being part of a child and family team is . . ."

Peggy answers, "Different ideas."

"Same purpose," Warren adds.

"We support one another," says Mr. Camelini.

"I'm a member of this child and family team because . . ."

"I want to help the child," says Mr. Stewart.

"I love Kevin," says Warren.

Mrs. Stewart moves off task at that comment. "I think we all love Kevin, that's a given. But how can we convince him of that? He'll get right in my face and say—you don't love me. You've never loved me. You know how that makes me feel?" Her tone is sincere, and her voice is loud and animated. Mr. Stewart answers her question by gesturing with his fingers to indicate an inch high.

"Give him a kiss on the forehead," Warren suggests.

"I do, and he slaps me," Mrs. Stewart shouts. "I give him a kiss, and he'll slap me. Or he'll shove me away." Her voice calms down, and she is crying.

Peggy says, "I want to address that when we're finished with the team building."

"Okay," I respond, ignoring her comment that indicates that she thinks this focus group is for team building. Maybe it is. "Let me finish, then we'll come back. This team being strengths-based means . . ."

Nancy answers, "Strengths-based is focusing on some things that Kevin is doing well or succeeding in, or strengths we have as a team. Strength in the family."

I notice that all team members are sitting forward except for Mrs. Stewart, who has begun leaning back against the back of her chair. She's no longer crying.

Peggy answers. "It means that we focus as much as we can on the positive and where we can go, and we really try not to get marred down in all the negative."

Mrs. Stewart suddenly steps out of the room. We continue without commenting.

"To this team, empowerment means . . ."

It takes a few minutes for someone to answer.

Mr. Camelini answers. "We have the authority to do, collectively, whatever needs to be done."

Jane adds, "That's the ultimate that we want Mom and Dad to have—empowerment. Give them the tools needed to be able to control him on his own without us; eventually he's under their control."

Mrs. Stewart returns to the room, wiping her eyes.

"To this team, having hope means . . ."

Nancy answers: "That's a thing that we all have. We form together as a team in the hope that our coming together with our different strengths, and areas of experience, and knowledge, and what the family has, that we can all come up with some ideas to help Kevin and to help the family."

Mrs. Stewart takes a sip of her Coke.

"To this team, family-centered means . . ."

"Getting things back to a fairly normal level. Where everything is pretty well in a nice circle instead of all tangled up," Mrs. Stewart says.

"To this team, individualized care means . . ."

Mrs. Stewart answers, "Getting the child what he needs, regardless of what it may be."

"To this team, being a team means . . ."

Warren responds, "Working together, to improve Kevin."

"To this team the future is . . ."

"Now." Warren says emphatically.

"It is," Peggy agrees.

Warren explains. "We build it now. It's now." He stands up and gets a Coke from the ice chest. "It's not tomorrow. Every day is a game. Every day we have to play the same game with Kevin. We can't play different games. So it's now."

"Okay, here's a good one. If this team were a car, what kind would it be?"

Mr. Stewart answers first. "Cadillac."

"Oh, I say a Mercedes, please," Mrs. Stewart says with a laugh. "Go high class!"

"I say a van so we can all get in," Nancy suggests.

"A semi!" Warren says.

Mrs. Stewart sits forward, her voice animated. "I got a better one. Ya'll ever watch 'Las Vegas,' the TV show? They have this nice long snow-white Hummer limousine. Big enough to carry all of us and then some." She gestures around the table to include everyone sitting there.

Jane says, "Protect us as we're driving."

"Yeah," Warren agrees. "Not moving too fast."

"The major thing contributing to this team's success is . . ."

"Working together," Mr. Stewart answers.

"Persistence," says Mr. Camelini.

"Determination," adds Mrs. Stewart.

"The major thing standing in the way of this team's success is . . ."

"Resources," says Peggy.

"Kevin's attitude," Mrs. Stewart adds. "At least at home. Here, if what ya'll say is correct, it's improving, but at home, it's going the other way."

"He'll be all right," Warren reassures her.

"I wish I could believe that."

"He'll be all right," Warren repeats.

"The major thing I require from this team is . . ."

"Honesty," says Jane.

"Exactly," says Mr. Stewart.

"This team provides me with . . ."

Warren adds, "Support."

Mr. Stewart adds, "Information."

"Different outlooks," says Jane.

"This team represents . . ."

"Hope," says Mrs. Stewart.

"This team's strengths are . . ."

"Us," says Mrs. Stewart.

"This group," Warren adds.

"I think we each bring a different skill to the table. Information," Peggy suggests.

Nancy adds, "We all have a common goal, which is to have things work at school and at home better for Kevin and his family. We all have a genuine hope that that happens."

"What's your vision for this team?"

They all look thoughtfully up at the ceiling for a minute.

Peggy sits forward and talks to the group. "I would like for us to have a meeting like this one day where both school staff and parents can say there's progress being made, we see a change."

"Just cleaning his room, without having to be told," Mrs. Stewart says.

Peggy looks her in the eye. "My goal would be even more simplistic than that, that he keeps his hands off you."

Mrs. Stewart nods. "That would be nice. I would like that. Keeping his hands off his brother in the middle of the night would be the next thing." Mr. Stewart and Mr. Camelini both nod in agreement.

"What's he doing?" Peggy asks her.

"I've been woke up at 3:00 in the morning because Gary's screaming. I mean actually screaming, like the people across the street when they're physically fighting. I'll come in there, Kevin will be on top of Gary—boom, boom, boom, boom, boom. Gary's trying to defend himself."

"How old is he?" Jane asks.

"Gary? He's only 11," Mrs. Stewart responds. "When Kevin gets on Gary, he always picks when Gary is vulnerable, like when he's asleep."

"He doesn't want to get nailed." Jane says with a laugh. "Does he hit him back?"

"Only to defend himself."

The Turning Point

"I'm going to be direct with you right now." Peggy leans in to Mrs. Stewart and looks her directly in the eye. She points to the table with her index finger for emphasis. She speaks slowly and deliberately. "I hope that you don't take offense, but if this doesn't stop, and you don't do whatever it takes, he's going to be abusing some woman."

"Kevin will kill somebody," Mrs. Stewart seems to agree.

"You're raising a spouse abuser, because of the way . . . ." Peggy doesn't get a chance to finish her sentence. Mrs. Stewart's voice raises to a scream. She stands up and faces up to Peggy. Her face is red.

She shouts, hands on her hips. "A what??"

"If we don't stop it, that's what's happening. If we don't stop it, somehow, no matter what method you take." Peggy pounds on the table.

"I'm raising a spouse abuser?" Mrs. Stewart yells. "I'm doing everything I can to keep that from happening, and you're telling me to my face that I'm raising a spouse abuser? When I do my best to get him . . ." Mrs. Stewart moves away from the table and paces around the room.

Alan has emerged from behind the camera. He escorts Mrs. Stewart back to her seat. He stands between her and Mr. Stewart. "I'd like to interrupt here, because what I'd like to do basically is follow up on this."

"I know what she means. I understand it," Mrs. Stewart says to Alan. She is gesturing dramatically with her hands.

Alan leans over the back of her chair. "So I have a few questions to ask. Would you answer them?" Alan asks her.

"Yeah."

"Okay. Let's finish what you're doing here, and then I'll ask my questions. Okay? Okay."

"Do you need me to stop?" I ask.

Peggy turns to Mrs. Stewart. "Sorry. I needed to—I just couldn't keep sitting here and not address this."

Mrs. Stewart is still reacting to Peggy's comment. "But I do everything I can to stop it."

Peggy responds. "I agree. I think it's beyond your ability to do."

I notice that they're speaking to each other more calmly now.

Alan stops them. "So let's stop there."

He turns back to me. "My questions to her will be about that, and forming a plan."

Nancy interjects to the team, "This is a focus group and not a team meeting, which is different for me; usually I jump in a whole lot more." I wonder if she is feeling defensive because Alan interjected into her team. I know I would be. I make a mental note to ask her about this later.

It doesn't occur to me that Alan interjected into my team meeting, also.

"That's fine. We've got time. If you want to discuss something you need to discuss, I'm okay with that," I respond to Alan.

Peggy responds to me. "I think that we need to go ahead and finish what we're supposed to be doing here and then we can talk about it."

Alan speaks to Peggy, "I'm going to follow up on the same direction you were going." Peggy pats Mrs. Stewart's leg and nods.

"All I had left was a kind of a wrap-up question to ask," I say.

"Why don't you ask that now?" Warren suggests.

"My wrap-up question is to go around the table and let everyone have a chance to say a last word, either something that I didn't ask that you want to say, or something you said that you want to say again," I offer.

Jane answers first. "Last word. It's come to a point where he needs more than just parental discipline. Because he's not accepting that. You have to go to the next step. How long are you going to wait? Something serious may happen. He has to be stopped now. We have to find something now, before it gets too serious."

Peggy speaks next. From the tone of her voice, I think she may be a little shell-shocked from her altercation with Mrs. Stewart. "I think this is a neat kid," she begins quietly. Mrs. Stewart turns her back on Peggy to reach for a Kleenex. Despite Peggy's attempts to make eye contact with her while speaking, Mrs. Stewart looks down at her lap. "My first experience with him was positive. I think that he has all kinds of potential, and I really hate to see it not be brought to the forefront. I think everybody on this team has that in mind. There's not a person sitting at this table that doesn't care about him. I think that's pretty good."

"I guess I think, thank goodness for the team." Nancy picks up the question, "We see a family and a child that's struggling. I have a great deal of confidence in this group of people. We have a dedicated teacher. When I think about how things were when Kevin first came to this school, and compare that with now—we're hearing there's a lot of improvement— that is very positive. The next thing we need to do is use what we've learned about Kevin—about what's working in one part of his life—and help it work in another part of his life. We need to support the family to do that."

Mrs. Stewart is wiping her eyes. Nancy continues, "You've seen a big behavior change. If we could take than into other areas of Kevin's life, that would really help."

Warren speaks next. "I see the future as now, and I think it's important that we deal with Kevin where he is now. He may be 14 years old, but we really need to try to figure out exactly what mental age level we're dealing with, and start communicating with him on his level, so that we don't miscommunicate with him. I'm really concerned about that because there's something inside of Kevin that has him confused and has him bottled up to the point where he acts out, he gets angry, he gets violent, he gets destructive. We need to try to figure out how we can get him past that point."

He speaks passionately and directly to each team member, making eye contact with each person as he looks around the table.

Mrs. Stewart cries quietly.

"There's something that has him at a block at that point where he won't move forward," Warren continues. "He's been trying and doing much better here at school. He's been having the same problems at home, so we need to try to figure out how to do this 24 hours a day, instead of just when he's in our company or when he's here at school. The rules here are a lot more formal and a lot stricter for him. Maybe we can start look- ing at some other issues at the house that have that same structure, so that he knows he has the same structure at home, at school, and on the bus."

At the other end of the table, Mrs. Stewart takes her husband's hand and speaks quietly to him. She gently rubs his back.

Warren continues. "That's why I'm concerned about that bus, because I know our kids get set off on the bus. The bus is a looser structure than the classroom. The bus driver's driving, he's not really paying that much attention. He might not have seen the initial problem that flipped Kevin off. There's a way kids can communicate with nonverbal communication. When these things take place, and with a kid like Kevin who's so talented and so intelligent, he sees these things a lot more than other kids see. If Kevin just gets up and reacts to it, and all they see is Kevin getting up, they can say only what they saw. That's one of my concerns. So I want to get Kevin a structure that's 24 hours, at home, on the bus, and at school, so he can continue to improve."

Mr. Camelini nods and takes his turn next. "I like what he said. I was thinking maybe his success here at school can extend into more of the day. The points I send home each day; I give his score and make comments. Maybe I could get comments back, like he had a good day yesterday, something to that effect, and I could set up some kind of reward, if he does have a good day at home, too." Several people nod in agreement. "But I'm concerned that he's abusing his brother and his mother." His voice gets animated. "No one has to live with abuse. In our society, no one has to—you don't have to be in an abusive situation."

Mr. Stewart wipes his beard and sits forward in his wheelchair. "I'd like to see Kevin continue to behave at school and get better. Also at home. With his brother and sister and friends. We've been asking for help, we've been getting it, and we appreciate it. We love Kevin, too. We want him to be more like his brother and sister and go by the rules."

Mrs. Stewart is fighting tears. "I just want him to behave. That's all."

"I'm done with all of my questions." I turn to Nancy. "Did you want to say something, or did you guys want to discuss some things?"

Nancy shakes her head. "I think that when we meet as a team again, what we need to start doing is coming up with some real specific things that might be of help."

Peggy asks, "Can I ask where we are about the program you were talking about in the home?"

Nancy answers, "They're saying they'll consider doing it, but I've been talking about possibly just buying it as a service out of our family budget."

Mrs. Stewart asks Nancy, "What about the mentor program? I see that on TV all the time. Isn't there somebody you know that would work with a mentor program that might help Kevin? You see it on TV all the time."

"Right. We talked about that. The question that she's talking about is maybe somebody to help work with you all about the behavior in the home, to structure your day from the time Kevin gets up, then when he gets home from school. Really specifically to help you all." I notice that Nancy really didn't address her question about the mentor program, and, I wonder, if they're going to pay for it anyway, why they don't go ahead and bring in the behavioral specialist she's referring to?

"Okay. I understand," Mrs. Stewart says, sitting back in her chair.

Alan pulls up a chair and joins the table. He speaks to Peggy. "To comment about some of those things, you did mention resources earlier. It's
very interesting and very true that our town has limited resources. But
there are some things that are available that are really not tied as much
to resources as just ways to be able to get them done. Part of that is that
mentoring thing, and part of that is the positive behavioral support. We
have to form a contract with them, and that's not going to be any time
soon." Oh. I wonder why. Bureaucracy delays again.

"What about therapy?" Peggy asks.

"Nora is Kevin's therapist," Mrs. Stewart answers.

"Has she done any sessions with both of you?"

"She sees Kevin every other month. It should be every month, but
how do we get Medicaid to pay for that? Before, Medicaid was paying for
every month."

Nancy enters the conversation. "Nora told me was that she wasn't
seeing Kevin even once a month. She would be glad to see him more than
that, but she said transportation is a problem. I reminded her that you all
now have bus passes, and transportation isn't a problem."

Mrs. Stewart responds, "I told her that. I can get Kevin there."

"Do you think it would be a good idea for Mrs. Stewart and Kevin to
have some sessions together?" Peggy asks, then turns to Mrs. Stewart and
says, "and I'm going to be real personal—if I were you, I would love to
have somebody I could talk to, because you've got a very difficult job that
you're doing."

Mrs. Stewart answers her directly. "I know I do, but there's one question I have to ask. I feel right now, you are putting all the blame for Kevin
on me. All of it. That's what it looks like." She starts crying again.

Warren jumps into the conversation. "No. What she said was because
of his behavior and actions toward you, it could potentially be a problem
in the future."

"Yes it could, but the only person she's talking about getting counseling other than Kevin is me."

"Because he's hurting you," Warren insists.

Mrs. Stewart responds, "What about his brother and sister?"

Peggy comes back with a quick answer. "That might not be a bad
idea."

Warren responds to her. "Maybe down the road, but right now he
needs to respect some authority."

Peggy turns to Mrs. Stewart. "He's got to stop hurting you."

Warren turns to Mrs. Stewart. "He's not respecting you. He won't
bother Mr. Stewart. He's bothering you. Because Kevin knows that

he can. Kevin knows that you've told that you don't bother Dad, you bother me."

Mrs. Stewart wipes her eyes. Her voice becomes loud and angry. "Only because of medical reasons; is that so damn wrong?" She is yelling.

Warren jumps into the conversation. "Hold it. Mrs. Stewart. The problem with that is this . . ."

Mrs. Stewart interrupts him. "You know, I'm about ready to give up. Everything I do is wrong!" she says, yelling and crying.

"It's not about you," Warren objects.

Mrs. Stewart doesn't seem to have heard him. "Everything I do is wrong!"

Warren responds, "It's about Kevin."

"I've got to protect everybody," Mrs. Stewart says tearfully. She puts her head in her hands.

Warren says quietly but forcefully, "I know, but it's about Kevin. Kevin needs the help. Kevin needs the help. So we have to help Kevin by keeping the same structure and keeping the same routine. If we don't, we're going to lose Kevin."

Mrs. Stewart looks up, sobbing. "Don't you think I know that? I'm awake every night thinking about that. Don't you think I think about that?"

Alan stands next to Mrs. Stewart. "Can I have five minutes outside with you?" She follows Alan into the hallway.

Conversation in the room is subdued.

Mr. Camelini speaks first. "I can understand why she feels the way she does, because she is the focus of his aggression."

There is a chorus of "yes" around the table.

Peggy agrees. "No doubt. I think she's got a very difficult job she's trying to do, and I think he cares about his mom. I really do. I think he very much loves his mother."

Warren nods. "There's no question. He will fight and die for her."

Peggy says passionately, "He can hurt her, she just can't allow that to happen."

Mr. Camelini turns to Mr. Stewart. "Does he bother you? She protects you."

"He does," Mr. Stewart answers. "He gets in my face. He hollers at me. He says 'I hate you, you're not my real daddy.' He puts his fists up."

"But he doesn't touch you," Mr. Camelini points out.

"I've had to push him away."

Warren chuckles. "He's done that to me. He's fearless."

Peggy laughs. "I will never forget with the school resource officer. I have never seen a student go up against him."

Jane laughs too. "I have. They end up in the dirt. Or being handcuffed and hauled off."

I'd Lose It All

Alan and Mrs. Stewart return. Mrs. Stewart sits in her chair looking down at her lap. Alan moves to the front of the room. "I need to write on something. Is it possible to write on the board?

I offer Alan my flip chart. Everyone except the Stewarts gets up and searches the room for markers and masking tape.

Alan turns to Warren. "First of all, it's nice working with you again. You and I haven't worked together in . . ."

"Five years," says Warren.

Alan speaks directly to Peggy. "I knew that what you said was from your heart, and it was about wanting everybody to be okay." It seems that his first order of business is to paraphrase and replay what was said. So everyone's voice is heard, maybe?

"Yeah. I'm real worried about her," Peggy responds.

I notice that everyone is settled down in their seats around the table.

"I know you are." Alan turns to Mrs. Stewart, who is looking down at her lap. "I think it was hard to hear what Peggy said. Mrs. Stewart has agreed to let me assist her to hear things as objectively as possible. I do believe that everybody around here is very concerned about one thing, and that's safety. I heard that all over. Safety was very, very critical. It sounds like Mrs. Stewart, your safety was pretty much right on the top."

"But mine doesn't matter," Mrs. Stewart insists.

"Yes, it does matter," Peggy argues. This is echoed by others.

Alan looks Mrs. Stewart in the eye. "The team believes that yours matters. Since this is a team, I think it's important to acknowledge that. Gary's safety was next, and then Karla's." He writes this on the flip chart.

Jane asks for clarification in a humorous way. "He doesn't pick on his sister? Or he gets so much pleasure out of his brother that he keeps whomping on him?"

Mrs. Stewart answers, "He don't pick on her as much."

Alan continues talking. "Now I think the other person's safety that's really important is Kevin's."

Mrs. Stewart responds, "As far as I'm concerned, Kevin's safety, Karla, Gary, and his," she nods toward Mr. Stewart, "are the important ones."

"Okay," says Alan. "But would this team be agreed that safety right now would be the number one issue, and that it's really important to come up with a safety plan?"

I notice Alan's team-based approach of getting team buy-in for any goals that they are setting. He also seems to be using the team's agreement to make a point to Mrs. Stewart.

Jane nods. "A safety issue is what got him to Washington High."

Alan looks at her. "So you would agree with that." Several people nod. "Okay. I got agreement from everybody that safety is a really important thing, and the plan is important. Okay. The team believes that Mom's safety is as important as Kevin's safety, is as important as Gary's safety."

He is momentarily interrupted by the intercom. The group looks up at the speaker. When the announcement is finished, attention turns back to Alan. He speaks directly to Mrs. Stewart.

"My first request is this," he says to her. "Could you in your heart work on the fact that you folks are equal right now as far as the need for safety?"

"I've tried," she responds in a low voice.

"So my request is continue to try. I'm not talking about doing anything, but I'm just saying in your heart, accepting that. That you're as important. So I want you to continue to work on that. Is that agreed on?"

"Yes."

"Good. 'Cause that's real important. We're talking about physical assault, and it sounds like the need is to stop the physical assault. Is everyone agreed on that? Okay. If I were to ask you all what it meant—we talked earlier about the police and about emergency commitment." Alan turns to Mr. Stewart. "If I were to ask the two of you what that meant—what does that mean?"

Mrs. Stewart answers. "I'd lose it all."

As Alan and Mrs. Stewart have what suddenly seems to be a private conversation, I notice that the rest of the group has changed their posture. Every person around the table is in "civil inattention" mode; sitting back in their chair, looking anywhere but at Alan or the Stewarts. They seem to have formed a bubble of privacy around Alan and Mrs. Stewart, but they are clearly listening intently to what they are saying. Except for Alan and Mrs. Stewart's conversation, you could hear a pin drop. I look down at the table, acutely aware that the tape recorder and video camera are still running. I wonder if anyone else remembers that now.

Alan continues. "So having the police come out and having him committed or sent down to the juvenile detention center means right now to you to lose everything."

"I have to protect the other children."

"Okay, so not just Kevin but the other two."

"I'd lose everything."

"So that's where you're coming from right now, is the fact that if you call those police folks out or we do an emergency commitment, then you lose everything."

"Child welfare would take the other two."

"If I were you I'd rather stay home and get slapped around."

"No, but I don't want to lose everything."

"But if I were you, if I thought I was going to lose everything, I'd rather stay home and get slapped around."

It seems to me that Alan is trying to show the group that Mrs. Stewart's behavior is not irrational, that it is, in fact, rational, given her situation.

Her response creates a buzz in the room. "I don't like it, but I really want six children. I cannot have three more. Nobody understands. Three of them I gave up for their own safety. Not me, but for them."

I can suddenly hear several faint side conversations around the table. Jane turns to me and whispers, "Did she say she gave up three kids?" I nod.

Alan ignores us. "So this fear of not calling the police goes deep and it goes way back."

"Yes."

"How old are those kids now?"

"Neal and Ray will be 20 and 19 this year."

"How old were they when you had to give them up?"

"Five and four."

"So that feeling still goes back a decade and a half."

"Yeah. But I did what was best for them." She wipes her eyes.

"I think you did."

"I did what was best for their sister, their newly born sister. I had her removed, to save her."

The team members are listening intently again.

"So when you don't call the police when Kevin's slapping people, it sounds like that's what's best for him. Based on the history of what's happened before. Am I understanding that right?"

"Something like that. With the way things are now, and I've seen how things are in the foster care system. They'd split them up. They'd send all three of them to different places. Nobody would care about Kevin's problems. Nobody would care. Call me wrong, call me crazy. I'm just trying to keep my family together. Using whatever means I have."

Alan confirms, "For some people it might be wrong, for some people it might be crazy, but I think that what you're trying to do is keep your family together. So it sounds like what we all have to do, to be able to help, is keep everybody safe. Both things have to happen. So there's fear of the system and the law."

I notice how Alan is confirming her view of the world. Reality confirmation support constructs a sense of humanness, respect, and understanding in a relationship, I think to myself.

"I'll tell you, my oldest three; it was all a lie. They said that I was a drug dealer and a drug user, and a prostitute. All three of those things—they had no proof of nothing. The day the three oldest were taken, they had came to the house two days before that. They all got clean bills of health. I'm not even allowed to go to the dependency hearing after they were taken. I have to find out from a third party that the very doctor who saw them two days before and gave them a clean bill of health, turns around and says all three are failure to thrive."

I noticed she's shifted to present tense, as if in her mind it's happening right now.

"So those things are just as clear to you today as they were before, aren't they?" Alan notices, too.

"It all is. People tell me I don't care about my kids. They're wrong. With Kevin—and before Kevin, Patti—I agonized for two months over what to do to keep her safe. I went to a friend. You wouldn't think a person like me would have a friend in what was then HRS, but she was my friend, 'cause she knew the truth, but she was all about the rules. I told her everything. I told her what had to be done. Not just to protect the child, but to protect me as well. It was done the way I said it had to be done. Or I wouldn't be sitting here. I'd be six feet under. If Patti and her father found out today that it was me, I'd still be there, six feet under, and there wouldn't be anything anybody could do. Not even him." She points to Mr. Stewart. "As much as he loves me, his physical condition would not prevent anything from happening. I know he feels bad about that, and he shouldn't, but I gave it a damn good fight. But I fear the system. That's why I haven't wanted to step over the line and go to the police. That's the only reason why. Because given my past history, even though none of what happened was my fault, child welfare would come in and take the other two. There's no open case, but with child welfare and my past record, they wouldn't need it."

Finally, someone else in the team finds their voice. Peggy asks, "I was wondering why child welfare would have to get involved?"

Mrs. Stewart answers in a loud voice, as if she is explaining things to a young child. "Because child welfare—every time a child is involved in a physical assault on an adult, child welfare has to be called. That is the law. That is the way that works. Whether it's the adult doing the physical abuse against the child or the child doing the physical abuse against the adult, child welfare has to be called because there is some concern why the child would do something against the adult."

I think back to other teams I've observed and heard about, and realize that she's right. She has every reason to be afraid, I think. I wonder if the other team members think so, too.

Alan continues, shifting his line of conversation to assignment mode. "So it sounds like one of the first things that needs to happen is we need to find out what will happen if the police are called. What are the ramifications, what are the things that happen after that?"

Several people murmur quietly. I hear someone say something about "legal."

Alan continues his assignments. "Peggy, would you agree to be the person that would find out about that?" He turns back to Mrs. Stewart. "It sounds like it's really important for you to know that if you make certain decisions about Kevin, that you're going to be together."

"But I won't."

"So it's going to be real important to help with this fear of the system. I agree."

Peggy has another suggestion. "What about getting some services from the domestic violence shelter? Because they're a really good advocate in making sure . . ."

Mrs. Stewart shakes her head adamantly. "That's about spousal abuse."

"It's for all kinds of family abuse. The reason I'm saying that is they are a safety net so that people don't get hurt by the system, too. They are good at that."

Alan jumps back in and writes on the flip chart. "All right. It sounds like we agree that some information's going to help. What's the next thing we need, to be able to help deal with the fear?"

Mrs. Stewart responds. "I don't want to lose Kevin no more than I want to lose the others."

"You're not going to lose them," Alan assures her. "Did I hear someone mention a lawyer a minute ago?"

Warren jumps in. "Yeah. That's what you need. A legal opinion."

Mrs. Stewart shakes her head. "I tried that. I tried that with my other kids. They were on HRS's side. Not mine. We don't care that you're not everything that they said you are. They took your kids. We are on their side. We don't care about you."

"When was this?"

"The last time was in '89, and that's when Neal and Ray were taken. I haven't bothered since, because the legal system is just not on the side of families like ours."

"So '89 feels like it was yesterday," Alan says quietly.

"Yes. Actually, if you want to go far back, go back to 1980."

"Twenty-four years."

"Yes. When Maria and her brother and sister were taken away from me. If it can be proved to me that I won't lose any of them from home—even Kevin—I'll do whatever is necessary, but I don't want to lose them."

Jane turns to me and whispers, "Has she lost two sets of kids?" I shrug my shoulders.

Alan responds to her. "I don't know—proof. That's a biggie. I think that there can be information, and I think there can be an opinion. As far as proof goes, I think you'll probably have to take it on faith."

"I don't have faith anymore."

"I know. But you have a team that supports you."

"But I'm still failing. If I wasn't, Kevin wouldn't be doing what he is. The physical violence. That's what I'm talking about." She's crying again.

Alan looks around the table. "I'm seeing people shaking their heads. The team doesn't believe you're failing. What would happen if we arranged a meeting with the Crisis Center and the juvenile detention center? The meeting would be for you to talk with these two folks. 'Cause if you called the police when Kevin was getting aggressive, he would go to one of these two places. It might be that if you knew what procedure was going on, and if you got an opinion from an attorney about what the current state of the law was as far as what they could do and what they can't do, then you could get closer to this."

Mrs. Stewart is sobbing now. Her voice is loud and impassioned. "Child welfare can do whatever they want. They can do whatever they damn well please. I've seen it on the news. They go into a home, they take out kids that aren't even being abused, and then the next day you see on the news a kid in foster care was beaten to death by the very people that child welfare expected to protect the child, and child welfare does nothing to them. They don't do nothing. How can I equate keeping everybody safe and doing what's right for Kevin?"

Alan nods. "All I'm asking you to do now, all the team's asking you to do . . ."

"I'm going to try," Mrs. Stewart interrupts.

"Take this step and let's see where we're at after that," Alan requests.

"I got no problem with that." She wipes her eyes.

Alan turns his attention to the rest of the table. "Now the next thing was, Peggy talked about the domestic violence shelter. They actually do a whole bunch of stuff. They actually do." He picks up his marker. "If these things could be done, could we say we're done with Step 1 of our safety plan?"

"Yes," Mrs. Stewart responds.

"Step 2 is what you're going to decide after we know this stuff," Alan says as he writes. He turns to Mrs. Stewart. "Who is the only person that can make that decision? You. Do you have our support?"

"Yes. I hope so," she responds hesitantly.

"Yes ma'am," Warren says forcefully.

Alan turns to Nancy. "So, you're going on vacation, and I get to take your place for this stuff while you're gone. I'll arrange a visit with the juvenile detention center, and I'll do that by Monday." He writes on the flip chart. "By next Monday, I'll have at least a set of phone calls if not a real meeting with the juvenile detention center."

Warren offers, "I can call an attorney friend of mine."

"Great, and the domestic violence shelter—Peggy, why don't you and Mrs. Stewart talk about that?"

"Now, what exactly will I ask the lawyer?" Warren clarifies.

"In a nutshell, we need help for Mrs. Stewart. She's afraid that if Kevin gets put in juvenile or the crisis center, she's afraid that child welfare is going to just step in and take them all." He turns to Mrs. Stewart. "That's very clear. I think we all understand why it's so hard for you to call the police at this point."

"That's what bothers me the most."

"I understand that. That makes sense. Let's do this, 'cause I feel like people can make good decisions with the most information possible and the most support." He turns to Warren. "What we need to know, is if he has to go to one of these programs, are they going to step in and take them all away?"

"Right. I understand. We'll help find those answers then you can make those decisions." Warren turns to Mrs. Stewart. "I'm a product of a foster home. I'm the oldest of seven. They ain't all bad," Warren discloses.

"Oh, I know that. I know that," she answers. I'm not convinced she does.

As I'm leaving the focus group, Warren and Nancy walk me to my car.

"I normally would have said more," Nancy says. "But this was your meeting, and I didn't want to interrupt what you were trying to do." Hmmm, I think. I had wondered why she hadn't jumped in. Perhaps she had wondered the same thing about me.

Warren comments, "I can't wait for you to tell us what this all means."

I respond, "I'm hoping you'll tell me."

They look at me quizzically.

It occurs to me that I don't know the Stewarts' first names. Whenever team members talk about them, they call them Mom or Dad, and when they talk to them, they call them Mr. or Mrs. What interesting commu-nication! Referring to her as Mom implies that they're relating to her in her social role rather than as an individual, and calling her Mrs. Stewart implies that they're thinking of her as Kevin's mother and Mr. Stewart's wife. Calling them by their roles or formal names certainly sets them apart from the rest of the team, who are all referred to on a first-name basis.

I think about how Alan's interjection into this meeting was a textbook example of a turning point. Turning points are critical points in time at which significant changes occur that dramatically redirect or change a system. When Alan took over the leadership of the meeting, because he introduced something different into the system, the system began operat-ing differently. It's not that the team was doing anything inherently wrong before then, but Alan modeled several important principles: assuming people are doing their best and that they are being logical, given their cir-cumstance; getting buy-in from the entire team on goals and directions; setting specific action steps with deadlines and assigned tasks. It appears that this resulted in all team members (including the Stewarts) feeling heard and, maybe, more hopeful.

CHAPTER 5

Union Gives Strength: Constructing Hope

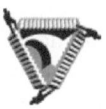

Undersized and Starved for Affection

A week later, I'm at the Stewarts' house. Alan's black sports car is already in their driveway when I arrive. He's sitting at what they use as their dining table, a dark wooden table that could be found at anyone's home, except that it's squeezed in their living room next to the front door, and the space is so tight that it's difficult for anyone except the children to get in or out. With effort, I slide onto the picnic-style bench next to the window. It's a beautiful spring day, and from my vantage point next to the sunlight, the house seems brighter, cleaner even, than when I saw it before. More hopeful, perhaps? I watch Alan and the Stewarts fill out paperwork as I try unsuccessfully to distract their tiny cat from chewing on the tie string hanging from my shirt. I make a mental note not to wear clothes with anything dangling from them the next time I visit the house. The cat is a tiny calico and looks like a kitten, but Mrs. Stewart tells me it's full grown.

"He's got six toes," she says, and, sure enough, he does! He's unrelenting in getting my attention and settles down when I pet him, but he refuses to let me stop. I look down as a very cute, tiny puppy rubs my leg.

"We just got him," Mrs. Stewart tells me as I attempt to pet the cat with one hand and the puppy with the other. It occurs to me that almost everything in this house is undersized and starved for affection. Despite the violence the family seems to exhibit, they have the most adorable, loving, affectionate animals. How bad can people be who have animals this affectionate?

Alan is helping the Stewarts go over their assistance budget.

"We need to get the bathtub repaired," Mrs. Stewart says. "I'm afraid someone will fall through the hole in it! Nancy keeps telling us there's no money in the budget to make the repairs!"

Alan looks at the budget. "I need to check on this to see if I can do it." He picks up the phone and calls his office. "We should be able to cover the repairs," he says when he gets off the phone. "See!" he points to a line item on the budget. "Let me make another call to see when we can get the check cut. Is it okay if we make it out to Lowe's?" The Stewarts nod. I am amazed at how quickly Alan makes things happen.

Alan is definitely a man in charge, but yet he and Mrs. Stewart are clearly working together. He hears her, listens to her, and acts on it. All right there at their kitchen table.

While they're working on the budget, the conversation digresses and returns. It seems as if everybody in the room has some level of ADHD, and I feel as if I'm watching a ping pong match. The conversation eventually moves in a direction, and things are getting done, but it's very hard to follow. Nobody seems able to focus on any one topic. They move from talking about the kids' needs, to creating a safety plan for the family, to the size of their house, to Kevin's medications.

"This is interesting," Alan says, as he looks over the paperwork. "Kevin is on two stimulant medications for asthma. Then, he's on two other stimulant medications for ADHD and depression. Do his different doctors know he's taking all these stimulant medications?"

Mrs. Stewart assures him that they do. The conversation moves back to the safety plan. I wonder if Kevin's medications, a crucial piece of information, I think, will be brought up again.

"I understand your concern that if you call 911 or do an emergency committal of Kevin for his violent behavior, that child welfare would get called in and you'd lose all your kids," Alan confirms. He leans in toward the Stewarts, listening closely as they sit around their table, working on a problem. Together.

"If child welfare came to this house, who knows what they would think!" Mrs. Stewart acknowledges. "They'd take the kids for sure! I don't want to lose my kids!" I hear passion in her voice as she says this, but I notice that she doesn't have an emotional outburst. It occurs to me that there's only one other time I haven't seen her have an emotional outburst—when I was interviewing her. I wonder if just giving her a chance to feel heard makes a difference to her emotionality.

"Let me show you the house," she offers. I decline, since I've seen it before, but Alan follows her from room to room. "Alan, look at her crafts!" I call out. "She's really talented!"

"We need space," Mrs. Stewart explains as she gives the tour. "There's no place to put things, for the kids to go without being in each other's faces. I could do my art and craft work if I had space to set up my sewing machine."

"She could sell her crafts, Alan!" I add. Several years ago, before I went to graduate school, I made and sold pottery and other crafts. My husband Jerry built me an art studio in our garage. I made only a few thousand dollars that year, but I had the time of my life doing it. I suddenly want that for her. A few thousand extra dollars could make a great different to the Stewarts.

Mrs. Stewart continues discussing her house as they walk back to the table. "We worked very hard to get another house. There must be some way to make it work, but nobody's been able to help us."

"They owe less than $4,000 on this house!" I interject. I know I'm supposed to be observing and not participating, but it's important to me that Alan knows that. I want him to fix things for her, right away.

I remember Nancy said that no bank would want to lend them money in their situation. Alan is listening thoughtfully as he sits down next to me. "I have a million things running around in my head right now," he says. "This is a safety issue." I wonder if he's trying to justify helping them. I'm excited as a glimmer of hope seems to break into their home.

Mrs. Stewart agrees. "If the boys weren't sharing a room, maybe they wouldn't be fighting as much." Alan nods as if this fact will make a difference in finding them funding. "We need to bring in a real estate person on the team. Someone who has the knowledge to do this sort of thing."

"Charlotte is a realtor," I whisper to Alan. Charlotte used to be a data collector for us who more recently did some work for the Center for Children and Families.

"Great idea!" Alan says to me. "So much for being an objective observer!" he comments with a smile, and I grin back. He turns to the Stewarts. "We need somebody who can help us to figure out who has funding to do this sort of thing."

Mrs. Stewart nods. "We just need somebody to loan us the money. We can sell this property. This place is almost paid off."

"This is a long-term goal," Alan cautions. "You know this is long term, right? We could be talking five years out!"

The Stewarts nod, but I'm not sure they really heard that. It occurs to me that this is the first hopeful thing about their housing situation I've heard anybody tell them. In one hour, he has made huge strides, in hopefulness at least.

What an interesting interaction, I think, as I get into my car. Alan exhibits strong active listening behaviors. He seems to do more immediate problem solving than anyone else who's working with this family. Does he hear them differently? When they express a need to him, he gets it done. Yet, he doesn't over-promise; he actually under-promises. He seems to instill hope by doing it—by moving and taking a step as large as he can. It seems there are many ways to construct hope. Alan gives people voice by helping them feel heard and then acting on what he hears. This confirms them as worthwhile people, validates their experience, acknowledges their ideas and suggestions, and moves them forward in positive ways.

Constructing Hope

On my way home, another man holds a sign at that same on-ramp. Ready for him, I hand him the dollar, and I'm amazed how incredibly grateful he is for my measly dollar. I'm relieved that no one behind me honks as I hold up traffic to give him the money. Isn't it interesting how much a person can appreciate a small amount of assistance? Just a little something to instill a sense of hope. It sure feels good to be able to help someone. I wonder if Alan feels the same way helping the Stewarts.

Continuing to Feel Supported

A few weeks later, Alan and I are in his office, working on a conference paper on a strengths-based approach to helping clients. We're supposed to be writing, but we're discussing my favorite topic right now, the Stewarts and my research project.

"How did your clinical background affect your work in systems of care?" I wonder.

"I always looked at people as individuals and formed relationships with the folks I worked with. But I saw them very clearly in terms of their diagnosis. This was either a kid with ADHD or this was a kid with depression."

"What's different in systems of care?"

"I still look at folks as folks, but now in terms of what their strengths are, what their needs are, what kinds of outcomes they're looking for."

"How do needs, strengths, and outcomes differ from pathology? Is it just different words?" I wonder.

"It's more than different words. If you're talking about therapy and pathology you're really just dealing with one domain—mental health—for interventions. Now we very clearly move beyond this kid's label or diagnosis. Now we think more about what the family's needs are on multiple life domains—housing, financial, recreational, safety—and how we can be of assistance with that. We sometimes put therapy and therapeutic interventions on a back burner until some of the other domains have been dealt with. Now, their family system is actually a point of intervention."

"But you were doing family therapy before."

"But now I look at it much more holistically," Alan explains.

"What was the impetus for your coming from behind the camera and changing your role?" I ask Alan, turning specifically to our last meeting.

"As I understood it, you needed a licensed therapist not on the team to intervene if things got to a point of crisis, or a point that was harmful to the family. When the school social worker very innocently—and on target—started talking about domestic violence, it was very clear that Mom reacted strongly to that. I think she was becoming disassociated from reality, and to continue that conversation without an intervention would be harmful to her."

"What was going on in your mind when that happened?" I wonder.

"Mom was disassociating like crazy, and it was time to stop that. 'Cause I didn't know her well enough to know how far it would go. Since then, I've learned from Nancy that she would have blown up and then regrouped, and it would have lasted about ten minutes. But at that point I wasn't sure."

"What were you intending to do?"

"Bring her back to today and alter her consciousness back into that. In some way interfere with her disassociated state. I did that because Nancy was getting ready to leave for London on vacation, and I knew that this situation was beginning to escalate. Kevin was settling down in school, and so the likelihood of it escalating back up at home was greater."

"Explain that to me," I ask.

"He has so much energy in him, he has to have an outlet. If he's doing better at school, he's going to explode someplace else, like at home, and Spring Break was coming up in a couple of weeks so he was going to be home all the time. Also, quite frankly, I was curious. I wondered, 'what's going on that he gets to beat you up but you won't fall?'"

"I guess it's appropriate for me to jump in and tell you what I think," I say. "What struck me is that the rest of the team seemed to be making the assumption that she did not have a good reason for refusing to call 911. You could feel the team believing that she was being resistant. The way you spoke to her communicated, 'I believe you have a good logical reason for doing this and I'd just like to know what it is.' You came at it from a different frame from the rest of the team."

Alan nods. "I did that on purpose, you're exactly right. I looked around the table and said to myself, 'these people think this lady's crazy, and it's crazy behavior, but there may be a good reason from her point of view, so let's find out.' Most folks that have had a traumatic past take on very unconventional types of opinions about certain interventions, processes, or of the world, but it's specifically due to the trauma they've experienced."

"I'm really curious," I say, "about your stepping in for Nancy. I have to say, Alan, that if it were me, and my boss had taken over a meeting in which I was in charge, I would be feeling pretty threatened. Yet, she says she's fine with that."

"Nancy and I go back many years," Alan says. "When she finished graduate school ten years ago, I provided her clinical supervision for her licensure, and I've continued to work with her as a clinical supervisor since then."

"I may be more neurotic than she is. I think that would make it worse for me," I respond.

Alan says, "We talked about it yesterday, and she told me that whenever I'm in the room with a family she's working with, she tends to look to me to intervene, and she's got to stop doing that. The two of us have to be aware of that. I don't want to do her job, because that may affect how the family perceives her."

I nod. "Let's go there, because I was going to ask that in a minute. How do you think the Stewarts perceive this situation—you're coming in and Nancy's leaving town, so you're going to do a couple sessions at home with them?"

Alan responds, "On one level I think they continue to feel supported, because it's not uncommon for me to take over for team leaders when they go on vacation."

I continue, "It strikes me that in the space of one focus group and one interaction with the family, they have been helped more by you in a couple hours than they were in four months before that. What's up with that?" I realize that I'm sounding critical of Nancy and the rest of the team. I feel a little guilty about that, but I'm really fascinated about what's happening.

Alan thinks for a minute and responds. "I think everybody has different identification with certain families. Sometimes you can identify with each other and bond right away, and other times that process takes a while. That's an intangible thing that I can never figure out."

I wonder, "Is it possible that the team leader can be so influenced by the system in which they're a part, that they can't change it because they're in it? Yet, perhaps somebody from outside the team can come in and make a very small change that makes huge changes in the system?"

Alan nods. "I think everybody came out of there with a much different impression of what motivates this lady than before, and a different way of being able to frame her behavior as something other than resistance. Now is she a pain in the butt? Yes. Is she irritating? Yes. It's hard to keep yourself focused and not let that influence what you're doing with people. It's hard for most people to do that. I've worked for a long, long time to get to a point where that doesn't happen."

"How do you do that?" I wonder. "How do you go into their home, look at their poverty, and the lack of cleanliness, and the unpleasant personality, and all the other things we could list? How do you see them differently?"

"I don't know that I'm seeing them differently," he responds. "I just can get to a point where I just don't pay attention to certain reactions that I have."

"What do you mean?" I ask.

"I just don't pay attention to my reactions," he explains. "Everything is a reaction—their reaction is a reaction, so every time somebody that you work with does something, you get a reaction to it. What you've got to do is basically say, 'okay, I'm not going to deal with that,' which I think allows you to be more present with the people you're working with."

I'm fascinated. "So what do you attend to? If you don't attend to your negative feelings, what do you attend to?"

"Them."

I recall how, when Alan and Mrs. Stewart were having their conversation in the time-out room, it was as if nobody else was in the room.

"The other day when I went with you to their home, what were you trying to do?" I ask.

"First, get rid of some damn bureaucratic stuff that we have to deal with, and then get to a safety plan. I went back on Monday and finished the safety planning," Alan adds.

"Which you said worked. What was in the safety plan?"

Alan responds, "We made more specific plans for visiting the crisis unit because we had determined that information would help them see the situation more rationally. My real intent is to never get to the point where they have to call the cops. However, the team needed to know that the safety issue was being dealt with, because that's a typical intervention, and for liability issues and reasons of general safety, we would have to talk about it."

"So, for the team's legal liability, they have to tell the family to call 911?"

"Yes, and for safety reasons, that's the typical response in this type of situation," Alan nods. "After that, I did a de-escalation procedure with each family member. I asked them each to come up with two behaviors that would make the family better and would decrease the arguing and combating. So each person, after 2½ hours, came up with—"

I interrupt. "A family full of ADHD."

Alan grins. "Oh boy! I tell you it was all over the place, but I like that kind of stuff."

"Yeah, after I had watched you with them, I felt like I had been watching a ping pong game," I say.

"Yeah, and those kids are just as active as the mom and dad, as far as that's concerned," he agrees.

"I haven't met the other two. I only know Kevin. He's just adorable," I say.

"Yeah, the other two are cute too," Alan says.

"They've got the cutest pets. I figure a family that has animals that affectionate can't be all bad."

"I don't think they are either," Alan says. "Quite frankly, I think they're just victims of their lives. I think all five of those people are very nice people."

"Mrs. Stewart needs to find a way to do her crafts and sell them. She could earn a living with those crafts," I hint.

"Probably." Alan returns to his story. "Anyway, so each of them came up with two behaviors, and most of them had to do with not being a pain in the butt for the other people. Mom of course had her blow-up."

"Did she?" I'm surprised.

"Of course," Alan responds.

"I had a theory that she wouldn't blow up with you. My theory was she felt heard by you, and she didn't feel the need to blow up."

"But I believe there's another reason why she blows up though. Not just one reason. She's got Post Traumatic Stress Disorder [PTSD] from the violence in her past, and every time you prick her on any of those PTSD issues, she's going to have an emotional reaction," he says.

"This is how she's communicating," I think out loud.

"She's actually letting me know that this is stuff that's painful, so it might be avoidance," Alan says. "I did with her what I do with a lot of people who are that way. I say, 'I'm about ready to say something that's going to be shocking or hard to swallow.'"

"Peggy did that in the focus group, did you notice?" I recall. "Right before she said what she said." Didn't help much, I think to myself.

"It's standard," Alan explains.

I shake my head. "I don't know if it would work with me. Jerry said that to me last night, 'I don't want to get you mad, but there's something I want to say to you,' and of course that made me mad, even before I heard what he said."

"In a therapeutic environment, it's respecting the fact that this is sensitive information and they may have a hard time dealing with it, and you're telling them that 'if you're not ready for it, we don't have to go there quite yet,'" Alan says.

"Giving permission to say 'I don't want to hear it now,'" I say.

"Yeah." Alan goes back to the story of the behavioral contract. "It was about her not yelling as much. Since she's enmeshed in this, she says, 'I don't know what else to do, don't know what else to do, don't know what else to do.' I asked her, 'would it be possible to work on not yelling as loudly,' and we talked about what loud meant. We worked up a plan in which each family member gets points for following their behaviors, and the family as a whole could get bonus points if everyone follows their behaviors, 'cause if you just do the kids it's not as powerful as if you do the whole family."

I'm fascinated. "So what did everyone do?"

"Almost exclusively it was about being less aggressive to the other person—not calling each other names, and not hitting. We did some bubble boundaries in which you can't go past the other person's boundaries except that you can turn off the bubble for hugs. They did great with it. I gave them a $25 gift certificate to Wal-Mart, because it's important for them to see that it's not just some esoteric kind of thing, there's actually a reward here."

"You gave it to them after the week was up?" I ask.

"No. I gave it to them at the beginning of the week, so they could see that it was there, but I asked Mom to hold onto it until I returned after Spring Break. They did nicely. Their violent behaviors had gone down a lot. So now my role with the family is to be their behavioral therapist. I want to go back and do more, since they seem to work real well with those behavioral approaches."

I'm impressed. "I wonder why is it, do you think, that there wasn't a safety plan in place before now, or why nobody had talked to them about getting another house? I'm just wondering why all this just came up when you were meeting with them. All of a sudden things are different, and I just wonder what's different, besides the different person working with them?"

"I don't know why we don't see certain things at a specific time," Alan responds thoughtfully. "I do know that there's a difference between talking and doing. It's really important to do."

"Is it a therapist orientation, do you think, to tend to do more talking than doing?" I ask.

"I think it is partially," Alan answers. "It may be that we talk, but not about focusing on the doing and the action, and we need to do that more. It may be that this team talked about safety previous to this time. It also could be that they were focusing on so many other things, because no matter what, you're still child-oriented, and this is the third school program this kid has been in."

I think back. "They were probably focusing on safety at school."

"They were dealing with issues at school," Alan says. "I know Nancy's energy went to being supportive of the school so he could settle down and stay there."

"Yeah," I remember. "Keep him on the bus, keep him from being kicked out."

"So that's where they focused. I don't think the team ever saw the level of violence in the home as being that critical a safety issue. It was more the way they are with each other as opposed to anything else. I think it's partially that that is just their culture, and it didn't hit the threshold."

Alan looks at his watch, so I ask my next question quickly. "I know you're in a hurry. Let me just throw out two other thoughts and get your reaction. One is an observation. It seems to me that the team has been operating in present or past tense. 'This is happening;' 'this did happen.' What I observed is that you started out in future tense. You were talking about getting a bigger house, and you said, 'this is going to be a long-range thing. It's not going to happen right now, but it will happen.' You were saying, 'we *will* get you the Lowe's gift certificate,' 'we *will* fix the bathroom.' You were operating in future tense. Deficits and strengths both seem to be rooted in the present and past, and I think that possibilities are rooted in the future. I'm hypothesizing that you moved them to possibilities in the future. Hope, too, resides in the future but is constructed in the present."

"That gets us back to that paper we're supposed to be writing today about strengths," Alan says, "and they're either talents, and then, I forget what the middle one was."

"Resiliency," I offer.

"Then the possibilities," Alan remembers.

"I'm thinking that the key might be the possibilities," I say.

"I don't know that I do that," Alan says.

"You did it in the home. I think you constructed hope for them. That's a thought I'm forming."

"If I did, I didn't do it consciously," he says.

I flip through the papers on my lap until I find my notes on hope.

"There's some recent research which has found that caregivers who are more hopeful are more satisfied with their children's mental health services in terms of their perceptions of the appropriateness of treatment, improvement in the child behavior and functioning improvement, and in family involvement in treatment" [Riley, Stromberg, & Clark, 2009], I say as I read. "In addition, 'hope' messages by providers promote caregiver strengths" [Kearney & Griffin, 2001].

Alan nods. "There's a psychological theory called 'hope theory' which says that hope is related to the ability to identify goals and dreams and motivate yourself to move toward those goals and dreams [Snyder, 2002]. In fact, I recall reading an article which said that, for some people, the action of pursuing goals leads to hopeful feelings and helps them cope with stress."

"Yes, some researchers talked about constructing a brighter future for patients through helping them reach their goals [Parkes & Freshwater, 2012]. And I've read that there's a relationship between hope and self-efficacy, perceived quality of life, mental health, and coping, among other things" [van Gestel-Timmermans, van den Bogaard, Brouwers, Herth, & van Nieuwenhuizen, 2010], I add.

I look back down at my notes. "Back to strengths. There seem to be eleven key ways in which strengths-based communication can be used to construct hope for a family," I say, reading from my notes. "Communication about child and family positive traits; child and family positive behaviors; child and family interests; child and family resilience; child and family dreams or possibilities; available family and team resources; borrowed strengths; past or historical strengths; environmental strengths; positive feelings, attitudes, and values; and hidden strengths. All of these construct hope when they're used to create possibility for the family and the team" [Davis, Mayo, Piecora, & Wimberley, 2012].

Alan nods.

"When you communicate about traits, you talk about things in which the child or family excel," I add. "The key to communicating about positive behaviors is to give specific behavioral examples of that, such as, last week you did this specific thing well. And it's helpful to use things a child is interested in doing that would move them in a positive direction."

"Yes, so in this team, examples of positive traits are Kevin's math ability or Mrs. Stewart's sewing skills," Alan says. "Mrs. Stewart is competent at seeking help for her family, and in communicating in a way in which her family's needs are heard."

I nod and look down at my notes. "Focusing on family or child competencies reminds everyone that they are greater than their problems, and it gives them a foundation on which to build goals and plans," I continue.

"Resiliencies tend to be thought of as personality traits that enable a child or family to have survived so far in the face of difficult life circumstances" [Dunst, Trivette, Davis, & Cornwell, 1994; Richardson, 2002].

"Resiliencies would include the persistence of Mrs. Stewart in obtaining help for her family," Alan adds.

"Exactly!" I say. "Communication about dreams or possibilities is also called "solution talk" in the literature [Berg & DeShazer, 1993; Fanger, 1993], referring to goals or dreams set in the future toward which the family and team are working. This type of strength-based communication uses imagery to show the family what they have to look forward to, or toward what they can accomplish [Fanger, 1993]. Possibilities also move the family out of a present-time focus, which is often laden with problems and deficits, into a future-time focus, which may be seen as a time of hope." I look up from my paper. "This would consist of a question like, 'What will it look like when things are better?' Possibilities focus the team away from problems or deficits and negative, destructive behaviors, toward positive, concrete alternatives. They move families out of an "either/or" orientation that limits their options, to a "both/and" orientation that opens up options and solutions [Lipchik, 1993]. Possibilities turn negatives into positives."

Alan nods. "A new home is a possibility for the Stewarts."

"Uh huh," I say, continuing to read. "Resources would include financial, time, and knowledge resources available to help the family and team achieve their goals. Mrs. Stewart's knowledge of the system is a resource. The assistance budget is a resource that you and Nancy provide, and psychological testing is a resource that the school provides. Other types of resources include environmental, food and clothing, medical, vocational, transportation, educational, recreational, emotional, cultural, and social resources" [Dunst et al., 1994].

Alan looks over my shoulder. "Strengths can be borrowed from another person, or by the strengths of the intervention or treatment itself" [Groopman, 2004]. He looks up at me. "Warren's intervention with Kevin's classroom was borrowed from the other work he had done in other schools, and the school staff's success in controlling Kevin's behavior was borrowed from their experience with other children at their school."

"Exactly," I affirm. "And past strengths are actually borrowed from the family's own history."

"The Stewarts can borrow from their past successes in getting help for their family," Alan says.

"Right! Environmental strengths are positive things in the environment, like the fact that the Stewarts have a home with a mother *and* a father at home. And the Stewart's desire to keep their family intact is a feeling, attitude, or value strength."

"What about hidden strengths?" Alan asks.

"Strengths that are, on the surface, deficits, but could be turned around into strengths. Kevin's aggressiveness could be a positive thing perhaps if he learned to channel it in a good direction." I pause, feeling excitement at how this concept is coming together. "Effective strengths give a family or team hope! So, communicating about talents gives hope because this show that the family is good at something that can be used to help them—it reminds everyone that the situation is not all bad or bleak. Communicating about a family's resiliency is helpful for the same reason. Reminding the team of possibilities gives hope because they orient the team into the hopeful future. Identifying resources in the team is also hopeful because that reminds everyone that they're not in this alone— that there are resources they can rely on for help. Borrowing strengths is hopeful because this also borrows hope—someone else could do this; this helped in another situation, therefore this will help here. Reminding them of past strengths is hopeful because that reminds everyone that the family accomplished something before, therefore they can do it again" [Davis, Mayo, Piecora, & Wimberley, 2012].

I close my notebook. "The other topic that I'm chewing on is the issue of empowerment. It's a question of—when is helping, helping? When is helping not helping, because it's disempowering? When is not helping, helping? When is not helping just plain not helping? I think there's a fine line there. I think everybody involved would have a different answer to that question, and their answer to that question would be reflected in how they're acting towards this family."

"There's a big clinical debate about that among therapists!" Alan says.

"Yeah, well, help is a two-edged sword," I say. "I've read that people with disabilities don't like to be helped because it's so disempowering [Braithwaite & Eckstein, 2003]. Receiving help can actually threaten a person's self-esteem, embarrass them, make them feel dependent, create a loss of control in the relationship, create feelings of inferiority, or create feelings of being patronized [Braithwaite & Eckstein, 2003]. Also, research [Ray, 1993] says that help creates power in a relationship. If I help you, then you owe me. Helping people sometimes reduces their power. Are you familiar with the concept of hegemony?"

Alan shakes his head.

"Sorry, jargon!" I say. "Hegemony refers to hidden power, and when you help someone, you can be reinforcing power positions of the person who is able to give help. Also, help can make the person being helped vulnerable to the people helping them."

"That makes sense," Alan says.

"Given all the difficulties with help, it's no wonder that this team has so many struggles with it" [Ray, 1993], I continue. "Since we haven't identified any way that the Stewarts can pay back the help, it puts the family in a one-down position in which they can't reciprocate. I've noticed that Mrs. Stewart has attempted to equalize this position by giving Nancy gifts of homemade crafts and flowers from her garden. I think that the team treads a fine line in giving Mrs. Stewart advice, as this kind of social support maintains their status quo and can potentially disregard Mrs. Stewart's point of view."

"Very interesting," Alan muses. "It seems that how much you tend to help a client depends on what your clinical orientation is. Also, I believe sometimes you've got to do things for people for a while, and then after that they need to do it for themselves."

I think to myself that by not helping the Stewarts move into a larger home until they feel they're ready, Alan and Nancy might think they're empowering the family, but I wonder if in fact they are disempowering them by keeping them "in their place" and holding them back. I wonder if this is a question of providing help at their current capability or perhaps stretching their capability. I also wonder if this is a question that doesn't really have an answer. Which of these options is empowering? Helping? Or, not helping? Which creates dependence? Which creates independence? Dunst and Trivette (1996) say that we enable people by "creating opportunities for competencies to be acquired or displayed as part of solving problems, meeting needs, or achieving aspirations" (p. 162). They suggest that people being helped must contribute to their own help if they are to acquire competencies, knowledge, and skills that empower them and strengthen their functioning. Helping people help themselves gives them a greater sense of control over their lives, while help that is paternalistic, patronizing, and unsolicited is disempowering and can be detrimental and debilitating for people (Dunst & Trivette, 1996). It can result in learned helplessness, a sense of incompetence and inadequacy, dependencies, low self-esteem and feelings of inferiority, and a sense of indebtedness and passivity.

"Well, helping the Stewarts is the reason the team exists," Alan suggests.

"Yes, and I think you struggle over how and when to best help them," I say. "And it's a fine line between doing it themselves, versus helping them do it, versus doing it for them. I think that's part of what we're seeing."

"Well, there's more than one way to help people," Alan says.

"That's true!" I agree. "Actually, according to the literature, there are at least ten kinds of ways you can support people." I count them on my fingers. "Helping or doing things for them; providing emotional support; providing information; providing material aid or giving them things or money; being a companion; providing love and affection; raising their self-esteem; connecting the person to others; giving non-judgmental listening support; or providing services" [Barbee & Cunningham, 1995; Cutrona & Suhr, 1992; Rosenfeld, Richman, & Bowen, 1998; Sherbourne & Stewart, 1991; Yu, Lee, & Woo, 2004].

"We're certainly helped the Stewarts in many of those ways," Alan says.

"Yes, and interestingly, when you're not able to provide Mrs. Stewart with the type of help she requests, you instead give her another type of social support, thus both helping and not helping at the same time."

"Really!" Alan says.

"For example," I continue, "I've seen Mrs. Stewart express a need for tangible support and receive emotional support instead. In the last focus group, she asked for listening and emotional support, and you all instead offered her informational and network support and then you provided her with emotional support, which calmed down her emotionality. What I wonder is, if you do that intentionally."

Alan shrugs. "It's definitely individualized, and for me that has a lot to do with a gut feeling of, 'okay, now it's time to back off.' Or, 'now it's time to say no, I ain't going to do this. It's your turn to do it.' I don't know that I know how to do it other than that's what my gut's telling me. Every human struggles with that."

I think of a conversation I had the day before with my sister-in-law Paula about my giving the dollar bills to the people on the side of the road.

"You can't coddle people," she said. "It's about tough love! Enabling them to continue depending on you is not helping them! They'll just take advantage of you! They need to learn how to be responsible for themselves!"

"What about compassion?" I countered. "How can I just let someone go without the basic necessities of life when I've been blessed with so much? I don't deserve what I've been given any more than they deserve what life has done to them!"

"They've got to hit rock bottom before they'll change their ways! You're just prolonging their suffering by preventing that from happening!"

I sigh. "I can't fix their problems for them, that's true. But, maybe I'm giving them hope when I help them out."

"You don't want to give them hope," she cautions. "Until they have no hope left, they won't seek help!"

The sad thing about the conversation is that we both were right. So, what's the answer? To help or not to help? I move my attention back to Alan.

"It's all very interesting," I say. "So your role on the team is moving toward, what? It looks to me like you're now on the team."

Alan smiles—or is it a grimace? "I'm now officially on the team, and Nancy has said yes and the family has said yes, and Nancy and I are going to try to work hard on role differential. She's fine with that."

"What's coming up with the family?"

"The tasks to handle in the next couple of weeks are reestablishing Nancy as the team leader and not me." That's very interesting, I think. So, he and Nancy did see a role conflict there. "How will you do that?" I ask.

"I'll stick specifically to what my assigned task is," Alan says, "which is to help the family with the behavioral plan."

I wonder if that is possible, but I just listen. "Uh huh."

Alan continues. "Oh, the thing I did last week was I took the kids out for ice cream for their bonus points, and that's also when I introduced them to Art, who's going to be the respite worker."

"Will he be a member of the team?" I need to make sure he signs a consent form.

Alan nods. "He'll be a member of the team."

"Not to make it all about me, but I have to ask, does he know about the research?"

Alan shakes his head.

"Would you or Nancy mind just mentioning to him about the research so when he sees me at a team meeting, he'll be expecting me?"

"I can do that," he agrees.

"You've got to do another safety plan," I prod.

"Yes, that's going to be part of their home behavior plan. I don't think that safety is the issue it appears to be. As a matter of fact, I want to start reframing that with everybody on the team, because to them this kid looks crazy, and he's not really crazy."

"What is he, then? What's wrong with him? Everyone has a different opinion." I ask.

"Clinically? I think the kid has Asperger's autism," Alan says.

"That's what Nancy thinks, too, but the neurological report didn't say that," I point out.

"Yeah, but has the neurologist been to any recent trainings on Asperger's?" Alan argues.

"The school people don't think that's what's wrong with him," I offer.

"Yeah, I know. So this kid probably can have many different labels at any point in time. He's probably just this neglected kid from an impoverished environment," Alan says.

"Interesting. You mention a good point: do the labels really matter?"

"They matter if you're going to use medication," Alan says.

Labels matter in other ways, too, I think. They reinforce the medical model, because the process of diagnosing privileges medical terminology and creates dependence on professionals who can label and then treat those labels. Gergen (1985) suggests that the behaviors themselves that are labeled as "mental illness" can be seen as social practice and social discourse, rather than mental states. Although I also think that labeling someone as "ill" may be somewhat more desirable than labeling them as "bad," "possessed," or "a witch"—all labels that have been used for mentally ill people earlier in our country's history—all of these labels still construct the other as deviant. I wonder if there is another way to see people whose behaviors do not fit into our society's criteria for "normal." I think about how this medicalization of behavior, especially for youth whose mental illness is behaviorally diagnosed, creates lifelong consequences for the child and his or her family. I wonder if, in some ways, a mental illness diagnosis is a punishment for a person's inability or unwillingness to be socialized to conform to society's norms and expectations (Foucault, 1965, 1995; Szasz, 1970, 1987).

"It also matters somewhat for the type of therapy that's used," Alan continues, bringing my attention back. "We also need to try to get his therapist on the team."

"Then you want to add a realtor, too, right?" I ask.

Alan nods. "Yes, we've got to help them with their house. They've got $4,000 dollars left on their mortgage!"

"Do you know what that says, Alan?" I interject. "They have paid off a $30,000 mortgage in 11 years! This family has more strengths than any of us are seeing."

"Yeah. In this economy—that's pretty good," he admits.

"When I figured that math out I was flabbergasted," I say. "When I interviewed Jane, she pointed out the strengths of the family."

"Oh, she's excellent at that," he says.

"When you think about it, as Jane pointed out to me, they're a two-parent family. They own their own home. The parents are interested in the kids. They're not blaming the system."

"They're willing to work," Alan nods and adds, "I think this team is in a trap. They're so overwhelmed they can't see much potential."

"Yes, they're part of the system," I say. "I think that the family looks so hopeless, they're creating hopelessness in the rest of the team. So, rather than the team pulling them up, I think they're dragging the team down. I don't mean that in a judgmental way," I add, as I listen to how negative that comment sounds.

"No, I agree with you, and I've seen that," Alan says. "I counted up the negative statements that Nancy made when we were discussing the family on Monday, and I said, 'Nancy, you said seven negative statements about this family, and they're all really emotionally laden,' and I left it at that."

"Interesting." I say. "The first time I met them I didn't like them. After I went to their home, I talked to my major professor and asked her, 'what do I do? I'm going to be writing about somebody I don't like, and not only that, but she's going to be reading this.' And, she's violent. One of the first things she said to me was she knew how to fight. She made her point."

"Same as a gorilla beats her chest, but they're never going to do anything. That's very defensive, doing stuff like that. Poor thing, she has to do that to exist in the world," Alan says.

I sit forward. "They're afraid of the world. The world is a scary place to them. When they go outside, their neighbors beat them up. Their house is like a cave." I pause. "But after I saw them through Jane's eyes and then your eyes, I've had a completely different picture of them as a family with strengths. I swear to you, when I was there recently, something was different. Their house looked cleaner than it was the first time I was there."

Alan nods. "It's better than it was."

"I'm starting to see hope for this family," I say.

"They've got a lot of strengths," he agrees. "If you're in this business for long enough dealing with really severe situations, burnout creeps in, and you've just got to constantly fight it. We even did it ourselves in the beginning, when we discussed this family in a staff meeting and said that we've got to be pretty limited with what our goals are, because they're hopeless."

"Wow. That's powerful." I am amazed at this confession.

"You're right. The family's depression sunk everybody else," Alan says.

I agree. "My first impression was—if I were a provider going into that home—I would avoid working with that family. I would do anything to avoid interaction with them," I confess.

"Everyone else who used to work with them very clearly said, 'Forget it. Just get the kid in school, it's fine.' But we said, 'No. We're not going to do that.'"

"But now there's a ray of hope," I say tentatively.

"Yeah, we've just got to do what we've got to do, and see where we'll go. 'Cause I have no clue," he says.

"I suspect families like that don't often have a future. I mean, from their point of view, the future's a pretty scary place," I offer.

"We can make it better," Alan says.

"Yeah," I agree. "What you're doing is painting a positive picture for them."

Alan nods. "Also, to be honest, what I really want is for this to stop in this generation, and I want those three kids to have a better life."

A better life. Is that so bad to want for someone? The question is, how can we best make that happen? Hope is one thing, but we've still got to take action. Like with my one-dollar bills.

Collecting Bills

Later that week, I'm eating lunch at Jason's Deli. Salad bar. My usual. "I'd like my change in one- dollar bills please, if that's possible." The cashier gives me a funny look but counts out a handful of dollars. I put them in my car. Collecting one-dollar bills for the guys standing on the side of the road has become a hobby.

Information Broker

My next interview is with Kevin's SED teacher, Mr. Camelini. He reminds me of my dad. He has the same white hair and mustache, kind smile, and quiet disposition. What he's doing teaching high school kids with SED, I have no idea. I'm interviewing him while the kids are outside playing basketball. I find out that this is a third career for him; he was a teacher once before, in the 60s, but had been in business since then.

"This must be a huge difference for you," I observe.

"When I taught in the 60s, some of my colleagues and I recognized that some students needed to be put in a special class, and we did that among ourselves and had success with them. If you have students reading at second-grade level in a seventh- or eighth-grade classroom, they get lost."

I glance at my watch. I have exactly 20 minutes before his class will return. "Tell me about the team from your point of view."

"It's only a team in the meetings," he answers cautiously. "I don't have any contact with Nancy outside the meetings. With Jane I do because she's here, especially if there's a discipline problem. Warren has been coming into my class on Mondays for about an hour, and he talks to the students about how they react to Kevin. The social worker, I don't have contact with her, either. She works up in the offices."

"At the last team meeting, there was a lot of conversation about Kevin doing better in school. What do you think has caused that?" I ask.

He answers thoughtfully. "The teacher's aide and I probably learned more how to deal with him. We wouldn't let him leave the classroom, so we deal with the problems in the portable. I think he's learned that we're serious, if we say we're going to do something we do it, and he doesn't run over us."

"That's wonderful," I respond.

"It is. I guess it's a matter of setting rules." He thinks for a minute and continues. "I don't have any contact with the team, except the daily point sheet that goes home. The parents sign it and send it back, but there are never any comments. At that meeting I suggested that we could incorporate his home behavior on our point sheet at school. I tried to set up some criteria, but I didn't ever get anywhere with it. I talked to Jane, and I sent it home with Kevin, and nothing ever came of it. I don't know if that's even a good idea, but it was an effort to extend our influence and our success that we're having at school into the home situation."

I nod. "I heard you mention it at the meeting. I thought it was a great idea. Alan is working with the family right now putting together a behavioral plan, and I wonder if he might incorporate that."

He looks surprised. "How often does he see them?"

"He went once right before Spring Break and had a great success. They were doing some kind of behavioral point system, and I wonder if you could put the two together." I notice that I seem to be serving as an "information broker" between team members—passing on information that provides each of them with hope or at least helps them to connect with the other team members. I continue. "You said you're really not having any interactions with the other members outside the team meetings, so I have to ask, do you think you guys are a team?"

Scratching his head, he ponders. "Based on the idea that I don't have contact with any of them except our people here, on a continuing basis, I don't think so. I don't think it's any more effective than what I would be doing in dealing with just the parents of the student."

"So you don't see any value, any advantage to these meetings?" I ask.

"Well," he hesitates.

"'Cause they take you out of your classroom," I guess.

He nods. "They do."

"So are they worth it?" I ask.

He responds. "Finding out more about Kevin and his family I guess has been very worthwhile. But those are things I could have found out just dealing with the family on my own. It's a severe case. He's very high maintenance, so learning something about the family life has been an advantage. Your question was, are we a team?"

"Uh huh."

"I don't know," he says. "I know I get frustrated in the meeting sometimes, because the same things come up all the time. He's abusive to his mother, and she doesn't want to do anything about it."

"What would you do differently in the team meetings?"

He thinks for a minute. "It might be of benefit to us, toward the end of the meeting, if whoever is in charge would just go team member to team member and indicate what steps they need to do before the next meeting, maybe kind of summarize it."

I think so, too. I've taught that in trainings I do on how to facilitate these types of meetings. Setting specific goals, then specific behavioral steps toward those goals, including assigned tasks with deadlines, is a positive, useful, and hopeful way to end team meetings. Check-ins with team members between meetings to share information and follow up on goals are also a good idea that moves the team forward, and creates a sense of "teamness."

I think it's interesting that Nancy hasn't been doing that. "That's a good idea. So everyone knows what's going on."

"Yeah," he says. "Specific things that the parents need to do. Specific things that I would need to do, or that Kevin might work on when he comes into the class. I don't know if Nancy has continued the relationship with them or not."

"I don't think you guys are a team yet," I note, "and I'm wondering— is it necessary for you to actually be a team? What would that mean for you to be more of a team?"

"I think it would be helpful for Kevin, yes, if we were a team. I think to really be considered a team, though, we would have to reach some sort of consensus on different issues, before our meeting ends. We haven't done that in the past, because when we thought we had reached consensus that the mother was going to call the police if she was abused again, she did not do it."

I nod.

"Also, can we be honest?" Mr. Camelini continues. "Can we sit in the meeting and be honest, and really say what we're thinking without getting anyone upset?"

"That's a really good point," I say. "It's hard to be a team without being able to be honest. What did you think about when Alan came from behind the camera and started working with the team? What was going through your mind?"

"Peggy was the brunt of the mother's anger and emotion," he says, "and I thought that was unfair, because she was just being honest. I thought Alan did a very good job of smoothing things down, getting to issues, digging in, and seeing what the problems are. That's when the information about another family came out."

"What does that mean to the team, to now know something you didn't know before?" I ask.

"It almost ties our hands, in a sense," he says. "We keep saying, 'you've got to call the police. If he abuses you, call the police.' She keeps saying 'I can't.' So, where do we go from there? It's almost like she's throwing up a roadblock. Was somebody going to work with her? I don't remember."

"Alan is now working with her," I say, "but you guys don't know that?"

"We haven't been told yet," he says.

I glance at my watch and decide to move to the next question. "Next question—do you think that the family is an equal member of the team, if there is a team?"

"That's hard to say," he responds. "All the other people are professionals. Parents, regardless of what their profession or their line of work is, they don't fit in that same group."

"Do you think the professionals are in a position of power over the parents in this team?" I wonder.

"Maybe that's why the mother gets emotional," he says. "I think they're probably overwhelmed. We probably put her in a defensive position."

I nod. "Do you think they have equal voice with the rest of the team?"

"I think they have the opportunity to, at least," Mr. Camelini responds.

"My observation is that you guys have incredible listening skills," I say. "Do you think that the family thinks you all think there's something wrong with them?"

"Yes."

"How do you think that affects the interactions in the team?"

"That puts them on the defensive."

"Is there any way around that?"

"No, I think there is something wrong with them. I think it's a dysfunctional family. I've never been to their house, but I can guess what it looks like," he says.

"It's probably worse than you could guess," I respond.

"Kevin's a mess," Mr. Camelini observes. "Kevin will come in here, and he rushes through his work, and it's sloppy and it's inaccurate, then he hands it in and he wants to do games. He'll start something, then he'll go to something else. He'll see someone else doing something else, and he leaves behind all of the stuff that he's worked with. He dresses messy. He smells like cigarette smoke, and the other students accuse him of smoking."

"It's in the house," I say.

"It must be."

"The house is black with smoke," I add.

He continues, "I know he's been given clothes from people here at school from time to time, and he'll wear them once and I don't see them again. I don't know if they lose them or they have an enormous dirty clothes pile."

"So what's going to happen to him? In the big picture."

"He will be a survivor."

"Really?" I'm a little surprised to hear him say that.

"Yes. Because he's scrappy. He's small, compared to my other students, but he doesn't put up with anything. He has a will, you can't squelch him, so I think he'll be fine. He can read and write well enough, and has enough academic skills that he'll get by. I don't think he'll be a college professor, but I think he'll be able to get employment and take care of himself."

A hidden strength, I think to myself. His "scrappiness" now gets him in trouble but in the future will let him "get by."

"That's encouraging," I say. "What's the team's hope for this family, do you think? What are you guys working toward?"

"To eliminate the violence and abuse at home," Mr. Camelini responds. "Things are pretty much under control at school, although at times he gets upset. He used to be picked on a lot. He's not picked on as much anymore."

"Why is that?" I wonder.

"There are other students that defend him," Mr. Camelini says.

"Really!" I'm surprised. "How did that come about?"

"I guess they see him as being at the bottom of the pecking order, the one that everybody can pick on, so some of the others defend him," he explains.

"Wow. That's incredible." What a change from the stories I heard at the beginning of the year. I wonder if Warren's interventions with the class have had anything to do with the change. I'm surprised Mr. Camelini doesn't mention that.

He continues. "The question was, what do we hope for? An end to the violence at home, and that he would be better assimilated at school. Maybe to learn how to dress a little better and take care of himself, be neater and cleaner. He has on cowboy boots today, and he walks into class and they start laughing. He doesn't care. That just goes over his head. I guess maybe to make him more sensitive to what's going on around him."

"So maybe a little bit better socialized. How are we are on time?" He nods, so I continue. "Do you think the family thinks the team has compassion for them?"

"Probably not. No, I don't, I would say no," Mr. Camelini says.

"Do you think the team does have compassion?" I ask.

"Absolutely."

"What do you think the team does that makes the family think they don't have compassion?" I ask.

"We're very honest. Very forward. Don't gloss over things. I would guess the mother is sitting there thinking these nasty people don't really understand. I'm just guessing," he says.

"Do you think the family thinks the team respects them?" I wonder.

"Will they look back and point to all of us and say, 'they really made a difference in his life?' I don't know. I would guess not."

"Do you think it would be better if the team members talked to one another more? If you got updates or had more frequent conversations?" I ask.

"The way we left the last meeting was kind of up in the air, you know. We said, 'call the police.' She said, 'I can't call the police' and gave the reasons why, so it was kind of a roadblock. I had the impression that Alan was going to be looking into some things so that if she did call the police there wouldn't be any consequences, so it would be the next team meeting before I found out."

"Are you curious? Would you like to know?" I ask.

"Absolutely. I would like to know, but it will be the next meeting before I find out. The same issue will come up," he says.

I open my mouth to ask another question, but we're abruptly interrupted by Kevin coming in the door. He gives me a hug when he sees me.

"Guess we're done!" I say to Mr. Camelini with a smile. "Maybe we can talk more later."

"Come any time," he says.

I get out of the portable as the kids rush in.

Something to Write About!

Interviewing my way through the team, I ask questions to find out their points of view of the team. A few days later, I sit in Peggy's portable in her small windowless office. It occurs to me that I really like her. She's a likeable woman, about my age, about my style. She's somebody that I could be friends with, I think. Her background includes social work in foster care, special-needs adoption, early childhood, and charter schools. She's now social worker for two high schools.

"Why this field?" I ask.

"I'm real people-oriented, so I knew I wanted to do something along those lines. Initially I was thinking of nursing, and I did a volunteer stint with geriatrics and that pretty much took care of that. Can't do smells! Blood's okay, but can't do smells."

I can relate.

"How long have you been doing this?" I wonder aloud.

"Twenty-three years," she answers.

I nod. "This family has a lot of experienced people helping them."

"I'm really amazed when we're all together in the same room," she agrees.

"Tell me about that."

"It's kind of interesting and comical, too," Peggy responds, "because there is a lot of experience and knowledge there, but such different personalities. It's just amazing to me."

"Tell me about the team meetings from your point of view."

She responds, "I am actually impressed with the family. That whole setting can be very intimidating, and I think that they handle it very well. Mrs. Stewart needs a lot of support, but she thrives on the attention she gets, and that helps her be a part of the team. Alan is amazing. Then I look at Mr. Camelini, who's trying to do every day what he needs to do for all those kids. Then Jane, she has such a diverse role in the school. She wears a zillion hats, and I think it's interesting to watch that whole process. This is a difficult family. I think it needs a team to balance things. What I am finding, too, is we all might get to a point differently, but we all get to the same point, and I think that's helpful for the family."

"What *is* the point?" I ask.

"Get the things said that need to be said, or to identify services, so, in that respect, I think we're on the same page. I don't think we have real diverse ideas on which way we should go. Different approaches maybe. I am impressed with the family, because it's hard to get with a group of professionals and hear things that you might not want to hear, or deal with things you don't want to deal with."

"What do you think it feels like to them?" I ask.

"I don't know that I could do it," she says. "There's so many of us in the meeting. I'm just way more private with my own self, so if I were in their position, I'd prefer to be working with one or two people."

I nod. "Given the privacy they have to give up to work with a team, is it worth it? Do you think the team approach is working?"

"I think overall, yes," Peggy says. "Everybody's hearing the same thing at the same time, which is real important."

"What is this team trying to do for this family? What's the goal?" I ask.

"That I'm not real clear on," Peggy admits, "because it's very client-led, so our goals shift from time to time. The biggest thing we're trying to do is support them in what they need to do to make things better for themselves. It might not always be what we want to do, but our main goal is to improve their life situation."

"Do you see that as the vision or mission?" I wonder.

"I think so," she responds. "I think it's to move them along a little bit. Their goals and our goals don't always match, but we get together. I hope we're going to have some change, even if it's in coping. If I didn't believe in that, I couldn't do what I do. I don't expect huge changes. I know the school is concerned about living situations and hygiene and lifestyle. My opinion is it would be ideal if they looked like this and did this, but that's their style of living, and it's not up to us to go in and make those changes for them. I would hope that we're going to improve their life in some way and help them cope. Also, I'd like them to take a little more responsibility for what they need to do for the child, especially in terms of mental health and parenting, 'cause I think their heart is there. I think they don't have a good knowledge of how to proceed."

I think about how, even though goals are, ideally, client led—or at least client focused—they can still be behaviorally and outcome specific. I also notice how, even in the face of fuzzy goals, the team has a strong overarching vision—to improve the life situation of the Stewarts. This is what is bringing them together. Having clearer goals to support that vision might move them—and the family—forward more effectively, I think.

"So is it the team's role to help them take more responsibility there, do you think?" I ask.

She answers, "I think the team is there to plan with them and set some goals and get some resources for them. I think we all bring our own little agenda as to what we'd like to see happen, but as a whole team, I would say we're there for goal-setting and helping them to get there."

"I don't have a social work background," I say, "so feel free to tell me this isn't the way I should be thinking. But in observing this team and this family, I have felt very frustrated that things aren't moving forward more quickly. I've struggled with what I think is a key question here: When is helping not helping? When is not helping actually helping, or when is not helping just plain not helping? I think it's a fine line, and I wonder if you all are dancing around it. Sometimes I've thought, couldn't you do more to push things along, but then I've thought, well, maybe you're trying to empower the family by not doing more. Sometimes I just want something to happen. Is that just me?" I'm very conscious of my desire not to sound too negative about the team. I'm interested in what she has to say.

"No," she responds, "I think you're right, because I know that we're on a team—for instance, when I became very confrontational with the family in our last team meeting."

"I was going to bring that up," I say with a smile.

"I realized quickly that I just did that in front of people, and in front of the team," Peggy says.

"Is that bad?"

"I felt it was not maybe the best thing to do in respect to the family," she responds.

"Oh, privacy, public," I say.

"Exactly," she says. "I think it needed to be done."

"What was going through your mind when that happened?"

Peggy laughs. "Honestly?"

I nod.

"I was thinking, 'oh my God, I've ruined her research!'"

I roar with laughter. "And I was thinking, 'thank God, now I've got something to write about!'" We both have a good laugh.

"What was your intention with saying what you said?"

"To get her attention. To really lay it out there. To really get a reaction, to make her own it."

"Which you did," I observe.

"It's what I would have done if I had been working with her one on one," she says.

"It was a turning point with the team," I comment.

"I put myself out there professionally though," she admits.

"In a good or a bad way?"

"Not in a good way," she responds. "It didn't feel good, because I do have a great respect for the personal dignity of people, regardless of who they are. They are people, and it bothered me that I had said that in front of people. I would have felt more comfortable saying what I said without other people witnessing it. So as soon as I said it, I thought 'oh God!' I realized as soon as I said it that I wouldn't be able to do damage control as well with the team sitting there. The team approach is very helpful in some ways, but I think in others, it may exact some change."

"What's your take on what Alan did?" I ask.

"It was textbook. I watched him do it, and I was like, 'oh my gosh! It's working!' First of all, he took the threat away, immediately, by telling them he was only going to ask questions. There was no opinion going to be stated, and the mother agreed to that, that he was only going to gather information. Then, the series of questions he asked, the way he got her to follow right down the road, I knew exactly when he got to the point where he was communicating to me why I got the reaction I got from her; it was just perfect. Truly. I was just so impressed."

"I also wonder if it was about voice," I share. "I think that she doesn't feel heard, and she gets loud to have voice. Alan let her feel heard. When you self-disclosed your feelings and concerns, you put yourself out there and made yourself vulnerable to her. One thing I've observed in my research is that vulnerability is often reciprocal. Often, if a provider appropriately self-discloses or shares personal thoughts or information with a client, the client is more likely to open up. If a provider appropriate shows vulnerability the client is more likely to be open to being vulnerable by making changes or trying new things. I wonder if it's the interpersonal connections that give clients support that enables them to reach out."

"Vulnerable is how I felt. I felt professionally vulnerable at that point," Peggy admits.

"I think that was the first time anybody on the team had let themselves, except for her, be vulnerable," I observe. "Vulnerability—opening yourself up like that—is the key to developing relationships, and I think she reciprocated. It took some intervention from Alan, but I think she made herself vulnerable by self-disclosing. Observing the energy in the room, I think it was a turning point as a team. Do you agree?"

"I'll be interested to see how she interacts with me at the next team meeting. I haven't interacted with her since then—there's not been a specific need to," she says.

"Uh huh."

She continues. "I would like to see her get some help. I think she needs to feel good, like she has a voice and power, because she really feels totally hopeless and out of control. That might even have been part of what motivated me, too, is to get her to take some power."

I nod. "I read some interesting research recently that said that if what people believe about the power they have to influence others matches their social role, they're more likely to speak up for themselves. If they're being asked to take on a role that doesn't fit the amount of power they believe to have, they're less likely to speak up. And if a person thinks she lacks power, she'll be less consistent in her behaviors" [Chen, Langner, & Mendoza-Denton, 2009; Kraus, Chen, & Keltner, 2011].

"What she wants is the for good of her child," she says, "but what she's doing is not getting it. She does have the power to do something about that, she just doesn't see it. I think it's going to be interesting. I think we'll either pull back, or something might get done," Peggy observes.

"So where is that fine line between helping and not helping and empowerment and disempowerment? How do you walk it?" I ask.

"For me, sometimes it takes me a long time to find the line. I tend to be a helper," Peggy explains. I immediately relate to this. I tend to have difficulty in knowing where to draw the line as well. I think of my previous job as a life coach. I suddenly remember that I had several clients who quit because I was pushing them too hard. I always blamed them for not being motivated to change. It occurs to me that maybe I should rethink how "helping" helps.

Peggy continues. "There's almost a gut feeling I have, it's like an instinct, I know if something isn't helping or if they're becoming dependent or taking advantage. I just know it."

"Where is the line with this family, do you think?" I ask.

"I think the family is going to have to take on more of the tasks involved. They're going to have to put their actions where their voice is, where their mouth is—what they're saying they want. Now is the time."

"You get knocked down so many times that it's just not worth getting up again," I observe.

"Yeah," she agrees. "I think she's just hanging in there. I don't think it's a lack of motivation, I really don't."

I move on to my next topic. "Do you think the team is a team? 'Cause I'm not sure I do."

Peggy laughs. "Yes and no. We have a common goal, to help the family in some way."

"Do you think it's necessary to be a team?" I ask.

"What I like about the team approach is that everybody hears the same thing at the same time and there's no miscommunication. The other thing I like about the team approach is that we concentrate on the big picture as much as we can. I think that's real helpful in the school system. I also like that the family hears some strengths, instead of negative, negative, negative. I don't think it would make a difference with this family if we were working with them individually or in a team. I don't think change is going to come quickly."

I start to ask my next question, but she continues. "My first contact with school personnel was that they were ready for me to move to a child welfare referral immediately."

"So you've come a long way, as a team," I observe.

"Definitely," she agrees. "From the bus driver on, they wanted me in that home. I told them as soon as I made the home visit, 'yeah, we could go that route, but then how's that going to help? This is a lifestyle.' The very first time I went out to the home, she started apologizing for how everything was. Then she wanted to show me the boys' room and kind of shift the blame on them, that they are the reason the house is the way it is. I said 'personally, this is just me, this would drive me crazy and I would just have to start tossing things out.' She said, 'I can't afford to do that.' As soon as she said that, there was no sense in even discussing that any further. That made me know exactly where she was, that this is a lifestyle. You see this with families with that mountain or hillbilly background. They are a rural farm family, and they're not going to throw anything away."

"Evidently not!" I say.

"So now, when he's really bad, we just send him over to the sink and say, wash up," she says. "If he has a new haircut I compliment him on it. Anything I see that's good, that's a change in his appearance, I compliment him on it. When he's dirty, we just say, 'go wash up.' So, I think we've come a long way, and I think the team approach is almost essential in the school system."

"Because?"

"Because it's not a system that recognizes that we don't have a perfect world with perfect kids with open minds. Because they are not teaching teachers family issues. We're not in the same world we lived in 20 years ago. I think in that respect, a team approach is essential."

"I was thinking last night," I say, "that I don't know if everyone has jelled into a team, but I think the school people have more jelled into a subteam. You all seem to communicate more frequently and be on the same page."

"I think that when the team members are all there," Peggy says, "it falls with the people that are doing it daily, and that's the family, the teacher, and the school. So the focus is more on that, but Nancy is very essential, because she structures the program and has the link to community resources. Warren is very important because he has a natural ability to communicate and work with families," Peggy responds. "In that respect, yes it's a team. We're definitely not all on the same page all the time. But we get there."

"So, what's the definition of a team?" I wonder.

"What does a team have to do or not do?" Peggy muses. "I think it's a team in a lot of ways more than other teams that I see. I think we're way more open."

"So what makes up a team? Openness? Honesty?" I ask.

"Yes. And safety," she answers.

"Safety?"

She nods. "It's the integrity of the team. No one's changing it, or manipulating it to suit their own agenda, that I can see. I think we're protective of the team and the goals and what we want to happen for that family, so there's unity in a way, even though it doesn't look like it. In other words, to my knowledge, I don't see sabotaging going on, and I have seen that before in other settings."

"That's what I love about these interviews," I say, "because you all tell me things that are a different way of looking at things. What do you think I should be seeing?"

Peggy thinks for a minute before answering. "I think it's the relationships that are forming, more than actually whether we're accomplishing the goal, at this point. I feel like there's more of a coming together."

I look at my watch and realize that over an hour has passed. "Let me ask you just a few last questions, 'cause I know I'm taking up your time. Do you think the team members make the family an equal member of the team?"

She thinks for a minute, looks up at me, and wrinkles her face. "I don't know. That's my yes and no look. Yes, I think because we verbally say we do, and eventually we do. I still don't think the family feels it, until a little ways down."

"Do you think they think so?" I ask.

She shrugs. "I hope so. I'm not sure they quite understand the direction the team could go, and isn't going, you know, with the whole power and child welfare kind of issues. But I hope they do. I don't know her exact experiences in the past, but if they've been such that no matter what she said, no matter what she did, this is what happened, I think she would have to see it at some level. We've been in and out of the home, and we've talked about our concerns with her, and what she is and isn't doing, and nothing's happened. Nobody's ripped her kids out of her house, and nobody's been banging at her door, so I would really hope she would see that. So in that respect, yeah, I do. I think eventually they feel like they're part of the team."

"So what about this power? How does that play out?" I ask.

"I definitely think that's shared. It's like a check and balance. No one can really take on that power. I don't think any of us would go against the team's wishes. I do think in that respect we're a team," she answers.

I ask my next question. "Do you think the team members make the family feel as though there's something wrong with them? Or do they make the family feel like they're normal?"

"I don't think that they can make the family feel totally normal, because that's not the case, and we would really be ineffective as a team if we didn't address issues. So I really hope that we're getting across that there are some problems here, in as nonthreatening a way as possible. I think her getting upset is just going to happen every single meeting. It's part of her personality. I'll be real surprised if we have a meeting all the way through during which somebody doesn't say something or she doesn't bring up something that causes her great distress."

"It's definitely her pattern at this point," I comment. "What about compassion? Do you feel like the family thinks the team has compassion for them?"

"I think it's moving in that direction," Peggy says.

"Is compassion something that's helpful?" I ask.

"With her, yes," she nods. "I think she really needs to feel cared for. I think if we can get that across to her, then I think she will be able to handle more criticisms."

"That's a good point. So criticism is easier to handle in a spirit of compassion." I say.

"Right," Peggy agrees.

Positive Changes

What an eye-opening conversation! After talking with Alan, Mr. Camelini, and Peggy about their reflections about the focus group, I'm very interested to see what happens in our next team meeting.

That next team meeting is rushed. "We only have 30 minutes for this meeting," Nancy announces to the group. "Mr. Camelini has to get back to class. I'll put the school stuff on the agenda first."

Most of the same team members are here, plus Alan, who is now a member of this team. Warren is missing. I'm disappointed; I had hoped to schedule our interview.

Nancy goes over her written agenda, then moves to the first item— strengths. "Mom is dependable. She returns my phone calls, she keeps appointments. Mr. Stewart shows concern."

Mrs. Stewart interjects, "He's taken on responsibilities of children that aren't his. A lot of men wouldn't do that." She turns to him and says with emotion, "you've got a heart as big as this entire state!"

The conversations turns to Kevin. "He really wants to change, but he doesn't know how," Mrs. Stewart says. "I'm not sure how to help him. Yesterday, he stopped Gary from arguing with him. He's trying to change."

"He can be very friendly," Nancy adds.

"He can be sweet as pie," Mrs. Stewart agrees.

"He's capable of making good choices," Nancy says.

"He's on Day 16 of Level 4," Jane adds. "That's the hard one," she says, acknowledging the progress he's made in his behavior at school.

"So, he's making some effort and we're seeing a change," Nancy affirms.

"If we make it all the way through Level 4, we start to think about a change in placement," Mr. Camelini suggests.

Nancy turns to Jane. "You mentioned on the phone that there are positive changes at school, but you also said that Kevin is see-sawing with Mr. Camelini."

"His grandfather died this week," Mrs. Stewart interrupts. "That could be affecting him. They used to be very close."

"I'm glad you told us that," Jane offers. "We'll keep that in mind."

The team expresses support for Mrs. Stewart, whose step-father was the grandfather that died.

"What's working for you?" Nancy asks Mr. Camelini.

"Our staff is now on the same page with his behavior," Mr. Camelini responds. "The plan is really working. Firmness and consistency. We refuse to let him leave the classroom."

"Yesterday he was playing football with another kid nine times his size. It was great!" Jane mentions.

"He used to feel out of place," Nancy says.

Mr. Camelini comments, "Not anymore. He's making great progress in socialization and getting along with the other students."

"It used to be that unstructured time was a problem," Nancy adds.

Mrs. Stewart interjects. "At home, during unstructured time, he plays checkers, chess, cards with Gary and Karla. It's the chores he has a problem with! Their arguing is good natured now!"

"That's music to my ears," affirms Alan. "Before, you were having a hard time seeing that."

"Last week, we went to the movies," Mrs. Stewart continues. "The kids saw *Scooby Doo*, and we saw *The Passion of the Christ*. Afterward, we discussed it with the kids. Kevin said, "if Jesus could do this for people he didn't know, I can do that for people I do know."

"Wow!" Nancy responds. "I can see his improved behavior is carrying over from school to home!"

Mrs. Stewart adds, "I'm very pleased. Last night, he agreed to take his bath!"

Jane nods. "He's growing up!" she says with a smile.

"With the bathroom renovated, looking the way it does now, they want to use it more!" Mrs. Stewart says with a smile. "He's still having problems keeping his room clean, though."

"Somebody had to give him a shower and clean clothes last week," Mr. Camelini interjects.

This dance between strengths, improvements, and deficits is interesting, I think, as I watch the team go back and forth.

"He still needs a goal to work on personal hygiene and grooming," Nancy says. "He's working with Alan on behavioral things. They can work on that." She writes this goal on the flip chart.

Mr. Stewart adds, "Alan's been helping us with the behavioral plan. When the kids get rewards, it's like flipping a switch. Last week we all went out for ice cream for getting points for good behavior. The behavior stuff is based on positives. He's trying to get as many points as he can to go to the store."

"He wants to buy something for me," Mrs. Stewart says.

"Let's talk about transportation issues," says Nancy. "You have $300 in the budget for your driver's license and driving lessons."

"I don't need lessons." She points to Mr. Stewart. "He can teach me."

Nancy moves to the flip chart. "What's our goal?" she asks Mrs. Stewart.

"Learning how to drive and having a license," Mrs. Stewart responds.

"What time frame?" Nancy asks.

"By mid-summer I could have my driver's license."

"I'm having credit problems," Mrs. Stewart interjects as she describes a problem with a bill collector. The team offers lots of suggestions for dealing with the problem. Mrs. Stewart agrees to follow up on their suggestions. Nancy writes this as a goal on the flip chart.

"Mrs. Stewart will check her credit rating," Nancy says as she writes. "That will help us as we look at a loan to get a house."

I notice how Nancy is engaging Mrs. Stewart in setting behaviorally specific goals and action steps, with deadlines.

She turns to Alan. "Fill us in on the behavior plan."

"We had a safety concern with violence in the home, especially during Spring Break," Alan answers. "We set up a family behavior chart for each person. Everyone did great. We set up two rewards—ice cream with me, and a $5 allowance at the end of the week, if they got 60 percent achievement."

"Are you going to make it more permanent?" Jane asks.

"I would love it!" Mrs. Stewart responds. "The kids would love it!"

"We've increased positive behaviors," Alan notes.

"One reward I would love to give to them, even one time, more than anything else, is take them to Disney or Epcot," Mrs. Stewart says.

Jane turns to me. "I told you!" she says.

I nod and raise my eyebrows.

"They've never been there." Mrs. Stewart says. "They don't know what it's like." She reminisces about a time she went as a kid.

"Like a real family," Jane whispers to me.

"That's the kind of experience they don't have," Mrs. Stewart says, her voice breaking. "We used to go to the park. We used to have fun."

"We should all go," I whisper to Jane.

"Yeah!" she says.

"You should take the whole team to Disney!" I say to Alan, loud enough for the whole team to hear.

"Yeah!" Jane says enthusiastically. Alan ignores us.

Alan turns to Nancy. "Let's try to get discounts."

"Just to give the kids something to look forward to," Mrs. Stewart says, "to go to Disney."

Nancy hesitates. "With behavior changes, we do better with short-term changes. Most of us respond to short-term goals rather than long-term goals. They're two different things."

I wonder why she's trying to discourage the Disney trip.

Alan interjects. "We can set short and long-term rewards. We can have an overall goal that their home life will be safer. The main point is that the behaviors continue after the rewards are done."

Nancy turns to the team. "Should we renew the bus passes? This is a team, so I'd like the team's approval on that expenditure from the assistance budget."

There is no comment from the team, so Alan says, "We can provide the bus passes through mid-August." He turns to Mrs. Stewart. "The justification is, you're learning to drive, which increases your independence."

Mrs. Stewart responds. "So, I'll get the bus passes on Monday?"

"I don't know. I'll have to see when the checks come in."

"I'll check with you on Monday," Mrs. Stewart responds. I am amused at how Mrs. Stewart is holding Alan to his task.

"A friend of mine got us passes to Busch Gardens," Mrs. Stewart says.

"The kids loved it. They see their friends going to the beach and bowling, and they don't get to do anything like that," Mr. Stewart adds. "We feel bad that we can't take them places. We just don't have the money."

Alan turns to Mrs. Stewart. "I have a request for the next meeting. You've shown us your arts and crafts at your home. The rest of the team hasn't gotten to see that. Can you bring those in?"

"I can bring in my painted peacocks, even my embroidery," she offers.

I'm pleased that she's going to display her work for the team. Maybe someone will encourage her to begin selling it. As the meeting breaks up, Jane and I talk about our attempts at embroidery and knitting. I tell her about my disastrous attempt at crocheting a quilt, which ended up crooked.

"It's probably very beautiful, just creative!" Mrs. Stewart interjects with a big smile. It occurs to me that she can be a very nurturing person.

"Alan," I say as we walk out. "A trip to Disney with the whole team would be a great way for me to end my book!" I envision a group of us at the park, holding hands and walking into the sunset.

He laughs.

As People with Stories

A strange thing happens as I drive home from the meeting. As I pull off my exit, I find myself looking for a person on the side of the road. I'm surprised that I feel disappointment when no one is there. I realize that I've begun seeing these people on the side of the road as, well, people! They always have stories.

I think about the Bible passage that says, "whatever you do for the least of them, you do it for me."

"These people really are the face of God, aren't they?" I say to myself. Suddenly, I realize that giving them the dollar is more about me and my relationship with God than about helping them. I also realize that I'm beginning to see the Stewarts as people, like the rest of us, with strengths and problems, qualities that are endearing and ones that are irritating. Maybe it's more about relating and connecting than helping and fixing.

I can't wait to see what happens next.

CHAPTER 6

All Things Are Possible: Hoping and Helping

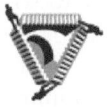

You're Influencing My Services

"Thursday at 9:00 A.M.," Alan confirms as he pops by my office. "We scheduled it for a time you're not teaching so you can be there. We'll be reviewing the behavioral plan with the family."

"See you then!" I say.

"I've just realized that the kids will be in school at that time, so I've decided to teach the parents how to administer the behavioral plan for the family themselves instead of my doing it," he says.

"You can reschedule it, if you need to," I offer. "Don't worry about whether or not I can be there."

"No. It'll be good to have the parents do it themselves," Alan insists. "So much for the independent researcher! Now you're influencing my services!" he adds with a wink.

"Uh oh!" I think.

"Oh, Alan," I stop him as he pauses at the doorway. "Did you hear about Warren? One of the researchers at the university is a friend of his. He's in St. Paul's Hospital with kidney failure! I heard he's waiting for a kidney transplant."

Alan looks as shocked as I was at the news. "No, I didn't know. I'll go by the hospital on my way back to the office."

Communicating Hope: An Ethnography of a Children's Mental Health Care Team by Christine S. Davis, 131–156 © 2013 Left Coast Press, Inc. All rights reserved.

I wonder if the team will send a card or visit him.

Thursday morning, the rain is pouring down in sheets as a river of water forms on the sides of the street. I'm a few minutes early at the Stewart's house, and hope the rain will slow before Alan gets here. I see someone peer out of their window at my car. I look up at the sky and see that the rain is showing no signs of stopping, so I open my car door. The rain soaks me before I get my umbrella open. I get out of the car and step in a huge lake-sized puddle. Water drenches my shoe. At least it's a hot day, so I should dry fairly quickly. I pull myself up on their front porch, trying not to slip on the wet ramp. I feel like I'm climbing into a tree house. When I open their front door, the strong smell of smoke hits my nostrils. I immediately notice that their windows are all closed, and even with two window air conditioning units running, the house smells moldy and dusty.

Their puppy runs to greet me. It's grown so much, I don't recognize it—it's twice the size it was the last time I was there. It jumps on me and nips on my fingers. "It's just being friendly," I tell myself, but I feel myself getting irritated when it won't leave me alone. Mrs. Stewart tries to get it to behave, but to little avail.

When Alan arrives, the dog finally tires and curls up next to us on the floor.

"Come see our bathroom!" Mrs. Stewart says to us. Alan and I look at their renovations.

Their workmanship looks good to me, but then what do I know about renovations? I'm impressed that they did all the work themselves. They put in a new bathtub, flooring, and a sink.

"Next time, you need to use Home Depot instead of Lowe's!" Mr. Stewart chides Alan. "Lowe's prices are more than twice what Home Depot's are!" From memory, he quotes exact prices—to the penny—from the two stores for a long list of supplies. I am impressed.

Alan pulls out his flip chart to go over the behavioral plan with the Stewarts. He begins listing the behavioral rewards.

"How about Disney World?" Mrs. Stewart suggests.

"Yeah!" I think to myself. "For the whole team!"

Mrs. Stewart mentions it two more times before Alan adds it to the flip chart under long-term goals. "It's important to have both short-term and long-term goals," he says.

"Put down a new house under there, too," Mrs. Stewart requests. She turns around and pulls out several homes magazines. "We want four to five bedrooms. Some land for the kids to play. There are lots of homes with some land out in Plant City!" She points to a picture. "See this one? $70,000. We could afford that! It's a fixer-upper, but we can fix things!"

Alan nods but doesn't say anything.

Mr. Stewart crosses the room and brings back a payment book. "We owe less than $3,000 on this place."

"A realtor told us we could sell this for $40,000," Mrs. Stewart adds.

"$35,000 would make a nice down payment," Alan comments.

The discussion moves back to Disney. "I could probably get passes," Alan says.

"We'd also need money for hotel and meals," Mrs. Stewart says thoughtfully. "We'd want to go for two days. To two parks. The kids have never been," she adds.

Alan puts a star next to Disney under long-term rewards. "If not this year, maybe next year," he says. They set other short-term rewards such as McDonalds and ice cream.

"How about some relationship-related rewards?" he asks. "What do the kids like to do? Play board games?"

Mr. Stewart shakes his head. "They like field trips, like to parks."

"How about the aquarium?" Mrs. Stewart asks.

I've lived here for three years and haven't been there myself, I think. I've got to get out more!

"The beach, movies!" she adds. "We love to go to the drive-in! It's cheap! I can't wait until the Van Helsing movie comes out!" she says.

"Oh, yeah, me too!" says Alan, who then launches into a discussion of several other vampire movies. I'm not a vampire movie fan, but Mrs. Stewart fills me in when she sees my blank look. "It's got Hugh Jackman in it," she says.

"Oh, I love him!" I say.

"Yeah, he's hot!" she says with a wink and then turns back to Alan for more vampire movie discussion.

"Do you remember that old TV show that used to be on?" she reminisces.

"Yeah, it always had horror movies on!" Alan remembers.

I sit back, watching, amused at how they connect over memories of television from 30 years ago.

"We need a new van," Mr. Stewart comments, when they return to business. "Ours has leaking seals."

"We're working on making a trade with a friend for a smaller van," Mrs. Stewart explains. Alan has no comment. They seem to have that situation under control.

They set behavioral goals, changing negative statements into positive ones: "Won't fight with siblings" becomes "will walk away when a fight breaks out."

I notice their strengths-based goals, stated specifically and measurably in terms of what will happen behaviorally rather than what they don't want to happen.

"Since we're meeting at a time when the kids aren't here, it's a good idea for you all to present this behavioral plan to them," Alan says to Mr. and Mrs. Stewart. "This way, you keep parental power and don't transfer it to me."

"That's a great idea," Mrs. Stewart says. "I had already mentioned that."

Alan looks at me with a wink. "Yeah, Cris's schedule influenced my intervention."

Mrs. Stewart jokingly jumps in to defend me. "Don't you pick on her!" she says. "Or I'll kick you, you know where!"

"You watch out, Alan," I say to him with a serious look. "I now have friends in high places in this house!"

"Come see the paintings I did," Mrs. Stewart says to me. "I'm thinking of selling them." I follow her into the kitchen where I try to ignore a roach and legions of flies. "I hate to sell them," she says, "but we really need the money."

"They're beautiful," I affirm, admiring a pastel-colored watercolor painting of flowers in a vase.

She points out some more of her crafts work.

"You could sell that, you know!" I comment. "At a flea market; you could make a lot of money!"

"Yeah, I could, but there's no space here to do the work. Even if I could, I have no money to buy start-up supplies. It's expensive to rent a booth at flea markets!"

Hmmm. I didn't know that. Couldn't Alan help with that? I think about hinting to Alan about that. One dilemma in helping people is deciding when helping is, in fact, helpful, or when holding back will be more helpful (in an empowering way) in the long run. I decide I've done enough hinting and should let Mrs. Stewart communicate that to him if she wants to.

"Here," she says, and hands me a gorgeous afghan. "It's for you. I made it myself."

It's bright, multicolored red, green, pink, blue, and yellow. "It's beautiful! But are you sure?" I don't know if it's ethical for me to accept a gift from her, but it would be rude to refuse it.

I'm reminded of reading that when people are on the "being helped" end of the helping relationship, they can feel worthless, disempowered, and helpless if they aren't able to reciprocate in some way. The rule of reciprocity is so strong in human nature that we feel a strong sense of obligation to reciprocate when another person has given us something or done something for us. We feel highly uncomfortable to be in a state of obligation, and we frown on other people who violate this "reciprocity rule." This is why asking for and accepting help is so difficult and looked down on. While people in helping professions often aren't used to receiving or accepting gifts from clients, doing so can represent a positive turning point in the relationship and a step in the direction of empowerment for the client.

I protest again, but she insists, so I take it. "I'll put it on our couch. I always get cold when I'm watching television." I'm touched that she would want to give me something, especially something she made, and it is beautiful. I wonder if I should wash it before I bring it into our house. I feel guilty thinking that.

We return to a conversation between Alan and Mr. Stewart. It seems that when he was in college, Alan worked night shift at a local mental hospital, and during that same time period, Mr. Stewart was an adolescent in-patient at the same hospital. They probably knew each other there.

"Yeah, I remember you!" Mr. Stewart says to Alan, with the excitement of someone who just saw an old classmate at a high school reunion.

"I wonder if you remember the old welfare worker we used to know," Mrs. Stewart reminisces. "Janice was her name. Tall, with dark hair."

Alan thinks for a minute. "I might have." I wonder if this was someone who worked with Mrs. Stewart's family when she was young.

"Here," Mrs. Stewart reaches behind her for a picture. It's an old picture of a baby in a metal frame. "This was my daughter. She'd be graduating from high school this year."

"She's beautiful," I say.

"My other kids would be 20 and 21 right now," she remembers. "They were adopted."

I notice that she keeps the kids' pictures out on the table next to her couch. I wonder if they've been there for the past 20 years.

When we leave, I'm relieved to see that the rain has stopped. Mrs. Stewart stops to pick a magnolia blossom off of a tree in her yard. "Here, this is for you," she says as she hands it to me. She hands Alan another one. "This is for Nancy." I breathe in the sweet fragrance as I navigate the puddle next to my car door.

There but for the Grace of God, Go I

At the off-ramp for my house, I'm surprised to find myself looking to see if there's someone with a sign standing there. I'm even more surprised to feel a sense of excitement that there is. I roll down my window and hand him one dollar. "Hey, how are you?" I ask.

"Where's the nearest drug store?" he responds.

"There's one at the next exit," I say, glancing at the light to make sure it's still red. "What do you need?"

"I just got out of hospital, I have stitches," he says. "I need to get a prescription filled."

"The next exit is five miles down. Can you walk that far?" I ask, wondering if it would be safe to offer to take him. I'm still weighing the danger when he assures me of his self-sufficiency. "I can get one of the truckers to take me," he says, pointing to the truck stop across the street. "How far off the exit is it?"

"Just a few yards. You can't miss it. Go east," I direct, mentally making sure I'm giving good directions, not one of my strong points.

The light changes. "Good luck!" I say.

"God bless you!" he responds.

I wonder what it would be like, just out of the hospital, with stitches, begging for money on the side of the road? I wonder if he got enough to buy his prescription. It occurs to me that most of us, regardless of how self-sufficient we think we are, are just one tragedy away from being in crisis mode.

Emotionally Insecure

He's the last roadside beggar I see for the rest of the month. I guess our unseasonably balmy spring makes it too hot to be hitchhiking.

A week and a half before the last day of school, we have the next team meeting immediately before our second focus group. The team decided that it would be easier to schedule one meeting time than two.

As a result, we're pressed for time. The meeting begins late, because Jane and Mr. Camelini are tied up with several fighting students. The police are called, and the entire school is in an uproar. Washington High has a brand new principal; this is his third day on the job. He is outside with Jane trying to settle down the students. Kids leave their classrooms to see what's going on. Kevin sees us meeting, and joins us.

The highlight of this meeting is a report by the school psychologist on Kevin.

"We did the Stanford-Binet, WISC 3," he says. I don't know what that means, but it sounds important. He reads the entire report, word for word, never looking up. Much of what he says doesn't make sense to me, but I can pick out parts. I wonder how much the family and Kevin understand. He reads in a monotone voice, throwing out jargon like weapons.

"Kevin is disheveled. Unkempt. Minimal concentration. Language appropriate. Friendly. Cooperative. Reynolds Intelligence Scales. Verbal

Intelligence. Nonverbal intelligence. Global functioning. Logical infer-
ences. Score 67. Verbal Index 88. Apply knowledge, low average. He
is very verbal. Nonverbal. Math, Reading, Spelling Score. Unexpectedly
high."

He pauses and looks up at the group. "That test must not be accurate,
too high for Kevin." He looks back down at his paper. "Up and down
there. Self-report for adolescent. Personal report. Indexes. Measure of
child's tendencies. Careless. Tends to hurry up. Critical items that war-
rant attention. Teacher rating scales. Acceptable. Critical items. Uses foul
language. Aggressive. Concrete orientations. Insecurity. Sub-intelligence.
Limited ego defense development. Will overreact. Doesn't realize that
most of his peers regard him in a negative manner. Doesn't see how he
brings this on himself. Does know right from wrong. Problem is ability to
control impulses. Emotionally insecure."

When he finishes, the entire table sits for a minute in silence, as if shell-
shocked.

Mrs. Stewart speaks first. "I'd like a copy of that. I want the doctor to
see that. He can't call me a liar now!" She turns to Kevin. "We'll show him
just how bad you are!"

Kevin begins kicking his chair and yelling.

Nancy addresses the psychologist. "Could you repeat the high scores
for Kevin's behalf? The ones you said were unexpected?" she asks.

"When we can get him settled down, he's able to do better," the psychologist responds. "We may want to look at it again in a year."

Nancy turns to Kevin. "When you settle down and put yourself to
work, you do good work." I notice she is making strong eye contact with
Kevin.

The psychologist interjects. "He can't handle a more demanding program than this one. We're setting him up for failure if we move him to a
more demanding program."

Peggy sits forward. "Is that on the table?" she asks. "This report shows
he meets criteria for SED. We can give him more services here."

"We need to do more testing," says the psychologist.

Kevin has been running around the room. He argues with Mrs. Stewart, who is trying to restrain him.

Nancy turns to him. "Your efforts have a lot to do with how things
are."

Mrs. Stewart adds, "He can do the right thing, he just needs to know
when."

Alan adds, "You see, we're all confused about what's going on inside
you."

"I think it's manipulative behavior," Mr. Camelini responds.

"We may have to do more testing," Alan suggests.

"This is the most restrictive setting we have," Peggy says. "We have to make sure we've tried everything else before thinking of moving him."

"If he tested differently, nothing would change for us here; we have both programs. A day program at another school may be another option," Jane adds.

Kevin is now running around the room, screaming.

Despite the best of intentions, we often get the behaviors we're constructing through communication, I think to myself.

Deeper into the Mind-Bending Universe

It takes about 20 minutes to get Kevin back to his classroom and settle the team down for the focus group. Even though Mrs. Stewart is still out with Kevin, I start the meeting quickly, as we only have 30 minutes before Alan and Nancy have to leave.

We start with the collage exercise.

"This is a collage that represents this team," I explain. "Your impressions of the team. I brought new magazines this time," I say, referring to the fact that they did the same exercise in the previous focus group.

"Did you say nude magazines?" Mr. Camelini asks incredulously.

"This is getting interesting!" says Margie, the Center for Children and Families' therapist who is helping videotape the meeting.

After some joking, the group settles down quickly to the task, looking through magazines, cutting, and gluing. Alan, Nancy, and Peggy help clear off lunch debris. Alan stands to reach magazines. Jane, Mr. Stewart, Mr. Camelini, Peggy, and Nancy sit comfortably as they look through magazines. Alan puts his magazine down and holds out his hand. Without a word being exchanged, from across the table, Peggy hands him scissors. There is some chatter about the magazine pictures.

Peggy asks, "Did we do this wrong last time so we have to do it again?"

"No!" I protest. "I thought it was so interesting, I wanted to do it again!"

Jane shows Peggy a picture.

Alan and Mr. Stewart compare pictures. Alan asks him, "You want me to put that in? Where do you want to put it?"

"We're trying to get in Kevin's mind!" Mr. Stewart responds.

"That's a good one!" Alan comments.

Jane studies a page. "45 Top Descriptions of Kids. All You Need to Know," she reads out loud.

"We should cut it out and paste it in your office," Peggy offers.

Mr. Camelini stands up and picks up a glue stick.

"This is more fun than taking pictures," Alan comments, referring to his videographer role in the last focus group.

I notice that Jane and Peggy are chatting. Mr. Camelini is working on his own, slightly away from the table.

The intercom blares, "The fire alarm will be going off. Please disregard it." Nobody seems to pay the message any attention. The fire alarm never does go off.

There is a knock at the door. Mrs. Stewart comes in, followed by Kevin. "See," she says. "Mr. Camelini is here! I will personally escort you back to class." She lets him get a soft drink, then they leave.

The door opens again, and the new principal, Mr. Casper, comes in. "I'm just coming to see how you're doing," he says to the room. He gives a hard look to the glue sticks and scissors. Mr. Camelini steps outside with him. When he returns, he does not rejoin the exercise but sits to the side grading papers while the rest of the team finishes the poster.

"You'd better introduce yourself to him after the meeting," Alan suggests to me. "Tell him what we're doing here."

Great.

I watch as a poster begins to form.

In the top center a headline says "Lifetime." There is a picture of a broken teacup with a band aid mending the break. In the center is a Lexus. I see a tossed salad. A picture of a room, neat as a pin, with hardwood floors and perfectly lined up files. A cartoon of a woman comforting a young boy, with a young girl crying in the background. "Hope" reads one headline. "Walls" in another. A mirror. A satellite. A young boy waiting for a ball to come down from the air. A picture of two boys in a classroom, raising their hands, with a headline "Education" and a subhead "Concern. Worldwide." Another headline, "Oh, I wish . . . ." Small girls playing soccer, great effort showing on their faces. Finally, a headline that reads: "Deeper into the Mind-Bending Universe Than You've Ever Been: A Guide in Plain English." That would make a good title for my book, I think.

"Okay," I say. "Explain to me what we've created. What are we saying about our team here?"

"In the center I put the Lexus," Mr. Camelini answers first. "When we first met, we didn't know one another, and we were pulling in different directions, but now we're a fine-tuned machine, moving along," he explains.

"Ooh," I respond. "You guys are a Lexus now. Cool. What else is here?"

"I put a salad," says Nancy, "'cause I think of this as healthy for us and for the family."

Jane and Mr. Stewart are flipping through magazines. Alan and Mr. Camelini watch them. Peggy gets up to get a soft drink.

Nancy leans forward and points to the poster. "This is a person doing his own thing and going his own way, and this is a group of people all working together to get to the goal." She looks at Alan and watches his reaction. He studies the board for a minute.

"Soccer players. Great," I comment.

"Get to the goal. That's neat," says Alan.

"Literally, get to the goal," I respond.

"Since we're close to the last day of school," Alan says, "I found this headline of concern about education. This other picture would represent a radar—we're still trying to listen very carefully and figure out what's going on. This other picture represents a goal that the family has, their house."

Mrs. Stewart comes back in the room and gets a drink. She looks over the poster and dabs glue under the corners of one of the pictures.

"What's the coffee cup?" I ask.

"It's broken. The band-aids are there to help," says Peggy.

"Anything else up there we haven't talked about?" I ask.

"Oh, I wish," says Jane, with feeling.

"Oh I wish," I repeat, momentarily confused; then I see the phrase on the poster. "Right."

"They wish for a lot of things," says Jane.

"There's the most important right there," adds Mrs. Stewart, pointing to the "Lifeline" headline.

"You can wish, you can hope," Jane adds.

"I put this because . . ." Mr. Stewart starts to say.

There is a knock on the door. Everyone looks up as Mr. Casper comes in and looks at Mr. Camelini. "When you're done, you're needed in the classroom."

"Okay, thank you," responds Mr. Camelini.

The conversation continues as if it wasn't interrupted. "In plain English," Mr. Stewart continues.

"Uh-huh, as a group, everybody, in plain English, where everybody can understand, and figure out what's on Kevin's mind," Mrs. Stewart says.

"That's great. That's appropriate," I say.

Mr. Stewart adds, "Kevin's mind is like outer space. There's so much there, but nobody knows what's in it."

"Exactly," agrees Mrs. Stewart.

"That's great. What's the cartoon?" I wonder.

"That reminded me of when Kevin was in here with us today," Nancy answers. "We all have a different perspective of him. This person on the team is going one way, another person is going another way, but we can all bring our perspective. Kevin can bring his and help us to understand some of the things he's thinking about. The team has a common goal from different perspectives." I notice that everyone is leaning forward, listening to her intently.

I glance at my watch and move quickly to my next question. "What's it like being a member of this team?"

"Complicated is the best word I can come up with," Mrs. Stewart responds. She is still standing, leaning against the back of her chair.

"In what way?" I ask.

"Well," she answers, looking around the table at everyone, "we're all trying to figure out what's driving Kevin, what his ultimate motives are, and so far we're coming up empty. It's hard to come up with the answers if you don't know the question."

Mr. Stewart leans back in his chair and puts his hands behind his head. "Yeah!" he responds.

Mrs. Stewart continues, "That's basically what it is. What's making Kevin do this, and then how do we solve it? It's like trying to put the cart before the horse," she explains in a serious tone, as if she's teaching a classroom of children.

"What was the question?" Peggy asks, as everyone laughs.

"What's it like being a member of this team?" I answer, then smile. "But you could answer any question you feel like answering."

"I got off from thinking about what she was saying," Peggy says. "One of the things that I get from the team is that so often, when I'm working with families, I feel like I'm by myself."

The door opens and the woman from the front office comes in and whispers something to Mrs. Stewart, who says "okay," then sits down in her chair.

Peggy continues: "Then I'm running around trying to connect everybody, and having everyone at the table really helps do that. We're all communicating at the same time and we all see what happens at the same time. For me, being part of the team really makes me feel less alone in what I'm trying to do."

The door opens again, then closes.

"I would mirror that. I agree," says Alan.

Mr. Stewart responds. "We agree. 'Cause a lot of times we feel like we're alone, trying to deal with this. But with the group, we don't feel so alone."

Mr. Casper returns and whispers to Jane for several seconds.

"I feel some frustration," says Mr. Camelini, seemingly ignoring the diversion at the other side of the table. "On one hand, it's great to have parents here, but as Mrs. Stewart said, I'm not sure how much progress we've made. When I'm in these meetings, I'm always torn; I want to be in the classroom."

"It's taking time away from your class," I acknowledge.

"Yes."

"We very much appreciate your . . ." Alan starts to say.

"Spending a lot more time with one student than I am with the others," Mr. Camelini interrupts.

Mrs. Stewart sits forward. "Like I said, Kevin's complicated. Finding out why he does what he does would make dealing with him so much easier, but we wind up with more questions than we have answers." Her hands are expressive and everyone is listening attentively to her. "One minute we think we know why Kevin does some of what he does and then the next minute that whole idea is shot out of the water because he's done something worse than what he had done before. That's what makes this whole situation complicated for everyone."

Peggy interrupts. "I do think it's frustrating because sometimes when we're trying to figure out why, we can get stuck there. One of the good things about a team is that if we do get stuck, there's always someone that can pull us out a little bit. We may never know why, but there's people, you included," she looks at Mrs. Stewart, "who know what works and doesn't work. So in that way I think a team approach is good. Sometimes it's frustrating because team involvement slows down the pace. So we have to have everybody on board from the beginning."

Alan nods. "It's one of those balance things. Sometimes, if you were just working on your own, it would be so much faster, 'cause it's just you doing it with the family, where with a team it does take longer to get everybody on board."

Peggy continues. "But who's to say that with the team approach we don't get where we're going, maybe a little slower, but maybe a little more lasting than you would with individuals?"

When the door opens again, Jane looks up and leaves the room. When Jane returns a moment later, she walks over to Mr. Camelini, shows him a paper, and steps back out of the room.

Mrs. Stewart jumps in. "They say too many cooks spoil the broth, but in this instance, I think the number of cooks actually makes the broth better, because they're each putting in a separate ingredient and not the same thing. No two people are going to put in the same idea, or look at something the same way."

"This is a good team," Alan says.

I ask my next question. "If you guys were making a movie of this team, what would the movie be like? Where would it take place?"

"I think the location we're at right now would be perfect," Mrs. Stewart answers. "The whole school environment."

"Documentary," Alan comments.

"Who would be there?" I ask.

"People like us," Mrs. Stewart says.

"Except Mr. Stewart would be called Julius Caesar," Alan interjects.

"Not hardly. I'm no Cleopatra!" Mrs. Stewart says.

"Demi Moore would play me," I say as everyone laughs. "What would be happening?"

"Exactly what is happening now," Mrs. Stewart answers. "Discussing what's the best way to help Kevin. Find out what's eating him, and what we can do to put a halt to it."

Nancy agrees. "I really like that idea. I was thinking the same thing. I think it would be real interesting if we were making a movie, to have this be part of it. Then, we'd follow Kevin through his whole day, starting at home, coming to school, going to class, riding the bus back home; brief little segments of each one, and then us as a team coming together with Kevin and talking about it." Everyone is nodding.

"Movies have to have a plot," I say. "What would the plot be?"

Peggy answers first. "The first thing that came to my mind was *The Bad News Bears*."

There's a knock on the door again, but no one comes in.

"That sounds like Kevin sometimes!" Mrs. Stewart says, laughing.

Peggy continues. "They're just a mess, with the whole sports theme, and the story is about the team and where they came from and where they went."

"The second one, *Breaking Training*," Mrs. Stewart adds.

"I haven't seen that one." Nancy says.

"They play baseball," Peggy explains. "Somebody winds up having to put a group of kids who can't do much of anything together to play ball, and they have nothing. They don't have uniforms. I don't remember who was in charge of them."

"Who *was* in charge of them?" Mrs. Stewart says thoughtfully.

"I want to say Rodney Dangerfield. No?" Peggy thinks.

"No, that was another soccer movie," Alan says. "It wasn't Walter Matthau, was it?" he asks.

"I think it was. Yeah, it was Walter Matthau," Mrs. Stewart confirms.

Peggy continues. "But anyway, through the course of the movie, they are a really good little ball playing team and they learn a lot about each other."

I ask: "Movies have to have dialogue. What would people be saying?"

Alan answers: "They wouldn't be saying just stuff about Kevin. 'Cause I don't think this is just all about Kevin. It's about your whole family," he says to the Stewarts.

Jane comes back into the room and returns to her seat at the table.

"It's about the entire family and the group itself," Mrs. Stewart says.

"How they interact with us," Mr. Stewart adds.

"I'm not even sure that Kevin would be the star," Alan thinks.

"Who's the star?" I ask.

Mrs. Stewart answers, "Actually, I think the entire team."

"An ensemble," Alan says. "Just like *Friends.*"

"But the entire team would be the actual stars of the movie," Mrs. Stewart says.

Peggy speaks up. "I was thinking of the show *24.* Every hour you see is an hour in the day, and there's 24 hours and there's 24 shows. It's a drama. I think it's in a hospital."

"He's a spy," Alan remembers.

"A spy. Even though we're not that exciting, I see it focusing on different parts of us, like Mr. Camelini in the classroom, you two at home, and individual therapy," Peggy says.

Mrs. Stewart interjects. "I can give a good example, too. Like *CSI.* They got two different cases going on at once, but they go back and forth between what one group is doing to solve this to what this second group is doing, and sometimes the two overlap. They become one case instead of two separate ones. Basically, that's exactly what's going on here. We have the team at school, then we have us at home, and when we come together at school, the two overlap into one. So it's a two-part thing. *CSI* actually fits the bill best because they have two cases going on at the same time."

"What would people be looking like, body language and facial expressions?" I ask.

"A variety," Peggy answers. "I don't think we could pin that down. Even when one person's talking, everybody's reacting differently. Sometimes I'm listening, sometimes I'm not. I might look like I'm listening, I might not be." Everyone laughs.

Mrs. Stewart says softly, "That's perfect. We have laughter. We all have concerns about Kevin, but in different ways."

The door opens. I am beginning to notice, with irritation, that it is squeaking more and more loudly every time it opens. Jane looks up at a teacher's aide, who says to her, "Have to go get Kevin." Jane jumps up and Mrs. Stewart puts her head in her hands.

Alan addresses her directly. "It would probably be a good idea, as much as possible, for you all to stay out of this one."

"Oh, I'm going to," she responds. "I'm not getting into this. I've got enough of a headache."

Alan reassures her: "He'll settle down after a bit."

"I did what I could," she says. "It's out of my hands now."

Jane returns and quietly says something to Peggy, who responds, "He only had one caffeine."

"Sometimes that's all you need," Jane says.

"Sometimes he don't need any caffeine to go off," Mrs. Stewart adds.

"Did he use that as his excuse that one day?" Jane asks Mr. Camelini.

"Yes."

"You had no running water and he had to drink soda," Jane says to the Stewarts.

"That was a bunch of bull," Mrs. Stewart responds.

I decide to move us along. "Let me ask you guys to complete some sentences. This is going to sound familiar 'cause we did it in the last meeting. I want to see how this team is changing over time. What I like about being part of this team is . . ."

Mr. Stewart answers first. "Everyone is trying to help."

Nancy says, "I feel like everybody is very interested, wants to do whatever they can, listens to everyone, tries to figure out how to help the family and the school."

Jane moves toward the door. She catches my eye and mouths "Got to go." I nod.

"From my perspective, it's good to get other people involved in what is a classroom problem," Mr. Camelini says.

"To this team, being strengths-based means . . ."

Mr. Camelini answers. "We have a variety of people here, involved in different ways."

Peggy adds, "It helps us to come off the negative and look at the positives. It's really easy to get into all the negatives, in any situation. That's human nature, so I think that the fact that the team is strengths-based helps a lot."

Mrs. Stewart rustles through her bag. I notice that she seems to do that a lot when Peggy is talking. I wonder if she's still angry with her from Peggy's comment in the earlier meeting.

Alan answers next. "For me, it's the struggle to define which strengths are going to be the ones to make the situation better."

"To this team, empowerment means . . ."

"Having what we need," Mr. Camelini says, "to do what we need to do."

"To this team, having hope means . . ."

"There is a solution we're working toward that's hopeful," Mr. Camelini says.

"As long as we have hope, we keep going," Peggy muses.

"Each time we meet, there's more information coming in. Hopefully we'll get to where we can make some recommendations," Mr. Camelini observes.

"Hope is motivation," Alan adds.

"To this team, family-centered means . . ."

"Instead of just the school," Peggy answers, "we're looking at what's going on with the family. We can get them and the teacher help and support, and we can merge all that. What I hope is that we'll get a lasting change. Something that will transcend whether he's at Washington or another school, whether you're living where you are now or not, something that will incorporate a life change for everybody."

"To this team, being a team means . . ."

"Working together, all pulling in the same direction, with the same focus," says Mr. Camelini.

"The major thing contributing to this team's success is . . ."

"The food," Mr. Camelini says, as he points to the spread of deli food I brought for lunch.

"Glad I could help," I say as everyone laughs.

The teacher's aide comes in the room again. She walks over to a refrigerator in the corner of the room and takes out a lunch box. The door squeaks as she goes back out.

"We're a very safe environment," Peggy says. "We're able to say what we think we need to say. It's not as though we freak out that Kevin's acting out. When Mom had her concerns and has become frustrated, we stayed together as a team with that. We just hang in there. I think it's safe. I think most everyone feels like they can say whatever they need to say."

We are momentarily interrupted by the intercom.

"The major thing standing in the way of this team's success is . . ."

"Apparently we need more information," Mr. Camelini says.

The door squeaks open again, then shuts.

"Not enough info, not enough time," Peggy says.

"The major thing I require or I need from this team is . . ."

There is a knock on the door. Margie, the therapist who is being videographer today, answers it. They speak briefly.

Mrs. Stewart answers my question. "Help for the whole family is what I would say. It's not just Kevin."

"It's not just Kevin," Mr. Stewart adds.

"It's not just Kevin that's affected by all of this, it's affected us as well," Mrs. Stewart repeats.

Jane comes back in the room and sits down next to the Stewarts.

"What's he up to?" Mrs. Stewart asks.

"Oh, just a little dickens," Jane answers with a smile that looks like a grimace.

"Oh, dear," Mrs. Stewart says.

"The major thing I need from this team . . ."

Alan answers. "I think we just need to continue to do what we're doing now, meeting together and continuing to participate in the process."

"I have one last question," I say. "I want you all to help me by being my research partners. The systems-of-care approach says that Alan, Nancy, Jane, Peggy, and Mr. Camelini aren't experts who impose things on the family, but instead we all work as a team together. Well, that's the way I want to see my research. Rather than my being the expert researcher coming in giving you my expert opinion, I want to respect your knowledge because you're living in the middle of this. I want to think of you as my research partners. So, my question is, what should I be looking at? Given that my topic is what's happening in a communications sense with this team, what questions should I be asking?"

Mrs. Stewart has several questions, unfortunately none of which are addressed by my research. "What triggers behavior of that nature? Nobody really understands what triggers ADHD, they've never fully found that. The doctor told me that. How do those triggers interact with the person's normal thinking? What do those triggers do to the emotional bonding that the person may have with someone else? Or with a group of others? Ultimately what would be the long-term cure for it?"

Alan finds a question that is more in line with my research. "How does a community-based team approach allow for the best functioning possible?"

"What questions should I be asking at the next focus group?" I ask.

Nancy responds. "One of the things I'd like to know is what people thought it was going to be like when we first came together as a team."

"What your expectations were," Peggy clarifies.

"If it's like that now, and where you'd like to see it go," Nancy continues.

Peggy asks: "What about, I don't know if this could be a question we could ask in a group setting, because it would be very revealing and we'd have to risk doing that, but I'm wondering if you would want to ask each of us to identify what we think our communication style is to begin with? Before we bring it into the team. Whether that changes, perhaps, how we normally would interact one on one, compared to how we would communicate in a group."

I wonder if she's still thinking about her personal interactions with Mrs. Stewart.

"If we're all going to work together, which we all are, why should there be what somebody would call secrets when we're all working for the same purpose anyway?" Mrs. Stewart argues.

"We're not talking about . . ." Peggy starts to say.

Mrs. Stewart interrupts her. "I don't mean secrets in that sense of the word . . ."

Peggy tries again. "Yeah, and I'm not talking about the team so much as I'm talking about her research. She wants to research how we communicate. There shouldn't be anything secret when we're sitting as a team, talking about what we're going to do as a team, to help the situation." She hesitates, and I feel sorry for her. Mrs. Stewart seems to be going out of her way to antagonize and fluster her. Peggy turns to me. "I understood you to be asking about the communication, not so much what's going on with Kevin or school or anything. So those are two different things."

Mrs. Stewart interjects: "If we don't talk about what is of importance to the team, then that would be a lack of communication."

Peggy looks confused. "I guess I misunderstand what she was asking."

Given that Peggy is now gun-shy about bringing up any sensitive topic with Mrs. Stewart, I think it's interesting that Mrs. Stewart is arguing against keeping secrets. I wonder if she's trying to give Peggy permission to say more to her. "It was a very open-ended question," I offer with a smile, trying to placate them.

Mrs. Stewart adds: "There's more to the entire group's communication than just what's going on with Kevin or with us or with the school. This particular group could be a model for the next series of children like Kevin who come along. They could use the example of what we have done as a basis to help some other children. I think that's what she might possibly be meaning."

"Sounds good," I say, trying to avoid being pigeonholed into one connotation. "It all sounds good."

Mrs. Stewart continues. "We could go on to help children that are worse than Kevin, 'cause no child with ADHD acts the same. One may have behavior and emotional problems. One may only have educational problems. Kevin unfortunately has all three, but others may have no emotional problems at all. So what we do in this group should help children who are worse than Kevin."

"What else should we do in the next focus group?" I ask.

Mrs. Stewart answers, "I have a suggestion. When we do the collage, why don't you put in your ideas?"

"Oh, okay!" I respond with a bit of surprise. From the beginning, I had wanted this research to be interactive, and I'm aware that it really hasn't been. This would give me a chance to introduce my ideas in a way that's more equal with the rest of the team.

"Because you've never done that," she adds.

"That's a good idea," Alan says.

Mrs. Stewart says, "I'm sure you have ideas that might be something we've never thought of."

Peggy adds, "I'd like to have feedback from what you're doing."

As much as I'm trying to move into a research *partner* role, here I am as expert again.

As I leave the meeting and walk over to the principal's office to explain my project to Mr. Casper, I realize that not one person has mentioned Warren or his absence. I wonder if they know he's ill. I wonder what that says about the team.

I think of how I've been called to the principal's office and thus called into account by the existing educational authority. Services for children are provided within the greater school system, under the system's rules and boundaries, and today's meeting illustrated that strongly, I think. I feel as though I'm back in third grade, in trouble for talking too much in class. These dominant hierarchies are hard to break (Gergen, 1999).

Those Dominant Hierarchies

That becomes apparent a month later, when I'm at the Stewart's. "Code enforcement's been out here," they tell me.

"We passed." Mr. Stewart says with pride.

I'm happy for them. "Congratulations!"

They have more good news.

"Kevin's been graduated. He's going to the tenth grade."

More congratulations! Things really seem to be looking up.

"Will he still have Mr. Camelini?" I know Kevin doesn't like changes.

"Mr. Camelini's gone," I'm told.

I'm shocked. "Where did he go?"

"Transferred. To a different school."

I remind myself that's the nature of these teams. From school year to school year, changes are made. I wonder how Kevin will handle the change.

They show me the family's behavioral plan for the past two weeks.

"Look at all those checkmarks! They've had almost no zero days," Mr. Stewart shows me with pride.

"This week is a little bit rough," Mrs. Stewart explains recent exceptions. "Art didn't come over on Friday like he promised." I remember that Art is the respite worker. I wonder what happened.

They Promised Me Help

After our meeting, I drive back to school in our usual afternoon rain shower. As I approach campus, I see what looks like a woman wrapped up in a poncho. She's holding a cardboard sign, illegible from the soaking rain. I reach for my purse to get out a dollar and realize that I don't have any. I think quickly, as I push aside strong feelings of regret and dismay. Instead, I grab a bottle of Kash 'n Karry water from my lunch bag.

"I'm sorry," I say. "I don't have any change. Will this help?"

I'm surprised she takes it so eagerly. "What time does the welfare office open tomorrow?" she asks. "It hasn't been open for the last two days because of the holiday, so I haven't gotten my money. They promised me help, but they haven't been open."

I don't know. I feel bad that I can't help her. "I'm sure they'll be open tomorrow," I say, and hope I'm right.

When I open my mail at home, a one dollar bill falls out of an envelope from a market research company. "Thanks, God!" I say. God always provides.

Behavioral Control

The daily rain showers blur one summer day into the next, and before I realize that much time has passed, it's the first team meeting of the new school year. "There's been a big improvement in Kevin's behavior at home and at school," Nancy summarizes. "He's had a big improvement academically."

"Our overall goal is family safety," Alan adds. "We're going to bring in a behavior specialist to enhance the behavior management plan we worked on this summer." He looks around the tables as he speaks, then focuses his gaze on Mrs. Stewart. "You've agreed to call the crisis center if necessary."

Mrs. Stewart nods with a grimace. "If it has to be done, it will be done," she responds.

Alan acknowledges her comment. "That's a real big leap."

"I hope it doesn't have to happen," she adds.

"I do, too," Alan agrees. "It's the right decision for safety."

Mrs. Stewart looks down. "I'm worried it might be my fault." I'm surprised that nobody picks up on the comment.

Alan looks around the table then back at Mrs. Stewart. "I'm glad the team agrees on the behavior specialist, and I'm glad you'll allow them to come into the home."

Addressing Mrs. Stewart, Nancy continues the conversation. "We have someone else that can help you address your space issues, how to organize and store things. This goes toward your overall bigger goal of a house. This is a little part of that, to help you do the best with what you have."

Mrs. Stewart interrupts. "I already have! I've run out of ideas."

Nancy nods. "They're a life skills program. They can give you ideas. I wish they could come to my home. They sit with you in your home and ask how they can be helpful to you."

Mrs. Stewart argues, "There's no way we can do anything else. We can't use the attic!"

Nancy responds, "Every family is different." Mrs. Stewart doesn't say anything, so she continues. "Are you willing to have them come in?"

Mrs. Stewart nods. "Anything they can do would be appreciated. I've run out of ideas!"

"I'll come out there with them," Nancy offers. "They'll just come out and talk."

Mrs. Stewart repeats, "I'm out of ideas."

Nancy continues to explain her suggestion. "They gave us a presentation. They had a lot of concrete suggestions."

Alan adds. "They'll get to know you and see how they can help." He turns to Mrs. Stewart. "That's a lot of people coming to your home. Let us know if it's overwhelming."

"They can come out!" Mrs. Stewart responds in an energetic voice. "If they can give me ideas so it doesn't look so cluttered, the more the merrier!"

Nancy continues with the agenda and turns to Mrs. Stewart. "There's a couple things you wanted me to bring up today. Transportation, medical, security, gas for cooking."

"Transportation first," Mrs. Stewart requests.

"You have an ongoing need for dependable transportation to places you need to go—shopping with the kids, medical transportation, family things, like the picnic with your kids this summer," Nancy begins.

"We're trying to sell the van," Mrs. Stewart explains to the group. "My sister is trying to help us with that. I want to get an older and smaller mini-van that I could drive." I remember seeing their old van in their driveway; it's a large 15-seat panel van. I rented one on 9/11 when I was stranded at the Atlanta airport; my feet barely reached the pedals, and Mrs. Stewart is smaller than I am. She continues: "One we could get his wheelchair in. I'm working on getting my license."

Nancy responds. "That's good. The bus passes we've been giving you aren't a long-term solution. You need something that you can do without us. There will be a time where we won't be involved in your life and transportation is a long-term goal for you."

Mr. Stewart interjects. "If you have three or more medical appointments a month, you can get free 30-day bus passes. But if you don't have three, you don't qualify. To go to the doctor last week, we had to save out $3 from our grocery money to pay for transportation."

Alan replies. "There may be a county program that could help with that, like a bus voucher."

"We can call for a Medicaid cab," Mr. Stewart explains. "But we have to call 24 hours in advance, so we can't do it for an emergency. They're a pain in the butt. Sometimes they don't show up, and if you're not done by a certain time, you don't get home. The bus is very reliable."

Alan nods. "But if we just keep giving you bus passes, we haven't helped you in the long run after we're no longer working with you."

"I'm afraid to drive the big van. I can get my driver's license right now, but I want to wait to drive the smaller van," says Mrs. Stewart.

"We can't afford gas for the big van," Mr. Stewart adds.

"So how about, we'll provide bus vouchers for three months," Alan offers. "During that time, you'll get your driver's license and we'll pay for an Auto Trader Magazine ad to sell the van."

Mrs. Stewart replies. "I'm willing to do whatever I have to do."

Nancy responds as she writes in her notes. "I think that's an excellent idea! To review, we're looking at selling the van, we're looking at an ad in Auto Trader, and we're looking at getting your driver's license."

Mrs. Stewart offers, "I could have my learner's permit by the next meeting, if I had the money to take the test."

"The money is in your budget," Alan says.

"Gas cards," Mr. Stewart adds.

"You may be eligible for county programs because of your disability," Alan says thoughtfully. "That would be long term. We'll find out what kinds of county assistance there is that doesn't go away."

"I should call the M.S. foundation to see what they have to offer," Mr. Stewart says.

"The next thing to talk about is your natural gas for your stove," Nancy begins. "You paid the bill twice for gas, but they cut it off because you paid cash and they said they didn't receive it."

Mrs. Stewart interrupts. "I want to explain!" She tries to grab the note paper from Nancy's hand. They tussle over the paper as they both laugh. Nancy wins.

"They've been making do on their barbecue grill," Nancy explains to the group. "They're doing a good job cooking on the grill."

"Until we ran out of charcoal," Mr. Stewart interrupts.

Mrs. Stewart has managed to get the paper away from Nancy. "I want to buy two 100-pound cylinders of gas. They're $150 each. They're pre-filled with gas. There's a $60 service charge, then after that, it's only $57 a tank to refill. That we can manage on our own. We on our own can manage that," she repeats, as she explains her plan in great detail. "We just need enough to get started. It's the setup we can't handle."

"Did y'all work out your relationship problems with the gas company?" Nancy asks.

Mrs. Stewart nods, and Nancy says, "Good job!"

"We're going to send them money orders from now on," Mrs. Stewart answers.

Jane asks a question, her first since I arrived. "Do you own this house?"

Nancy answers for her. "You've almost got it paid off!"

"In eight months it'll be paid off," Mrs. Stewart clarifies.

"There are three things," Alan begins at the same time that Jane says, "If you don't have money, Kevin doesn't need to have a Gatorade!"

Mrs. Stewart responds, "That was money he had earned."

"Yesterday he said that his coach gave him $20," Mr. Stewart adds.

Jane says loudly, "No!"

"Sometimes he steals," Mrs. Stewart notes. She tells a story about last Saturday. "He did work for his uncle. He was given $10. He got the dollar for the Gatorade from that."

"Two Gatorades and a cookie was $3," Jane says.

"I have no idea where he's getting it from," Mrs. Stewart responds.

"It sounds like this needs to be investigated," Alan suggests.

"Tell the teachers to lock up their purses," Mrs. Stewart suggests.

Alan repeats. "This needs to be addressed." He adds, "Let's table that for now."

Nancy takes over the lead. "We'll need to look into that." She turns to Alan. "There were three more points you wanted to cover."

Alan turns to Mrs. Stewart. "We need documents of two other estimates for the gas, because it's over $300. We need a written statement that you called two other places."

"I can do that!" Mrs. Stewart responds.

"This is a negotiation," Alan frames. "We can do this; it's in your budget. My next request is that you'll discuss with the life skills coach getting a checking account."

"We've got one!" Mrs. Stewart argues.

"Then, that you'll use it to pay these bills," Alan clarifies.

"He's just saying to discuss it," Nancy adds.

"Okay," Mrs. Stewart responds. "I'm easy to get along with. You know that," she directs to Alan.

"That's why I asked you," he responds.

"You wanted to change from the mental health center to Westside Mental Health," Nancy continues as she addresses Mrs. Stewart. "Do you still want to switch?"

"Last time I saw the doctor, I told him that Kevin was banging his head against the wall and threatening to kill himself. He ignored me. Maybe another place would be better."

Nancy responds. "I'm concerned that he's not listening to this."

"No facial expression, no verbal expression," Mr. Stewart adds.

Alan turns to the Stewarts. "There are three things you can do at the mental health center. You have a right to file a complaint. They have a process. They have to send it to a review committee. You can make a request for a change in psychiatrist. Do that first."

Mrs. Stewart nods. Nancy turns to her. "What did Alan say to do?"

"Put in a complaint, then request another psychiatrist," Mrs. Stewart responds.

"Who would you call?" Nancy asks her.

Mrs. Stewart shrugs. "I don't know."

"Call the main number," Alan instructs. "Say you want to file a complaint. We'll follow up on it, so call us as soon as you do it. You have the right to change."

"Is there anything else you want to cover?" Nancy asks the Stewarts.

Mrs. Stewart pulls out a brochure. "It's for a Medic Alert security system. They came by the house. Because of his disability. We can pay the $30 a month, we just need money for the installation."

Alan responds. "Can we wait for our next fiscal year, which starts next month? We can discuss it then after we see what our budget will be."

Across the table, Jane leans over to Nancy, "I need new slipcovers for my couch, too!" she whispers. I stifle a smile.

The Stewarts both nod their heads in response to Alan's request. It occurs to me that the way this assistance budget is set up, it almost feels as if the Stewarts are asking Santa Claus for presents.

Nancy interjects. "Let me go over what we talked about today. Academically, Kevin's showing a lot of improvement. His listening and his behavior with his peers are on track. Where's he getting the mystery money, that will be addressed by Jane and the school, and she'll communicate with you and me about that. There's the life skills program. The behavioral specialist will listen to the family and see what your needs are, how you would like things to be improved. Getting your driver's license. My part is to arrange the money; your part is to arrange the test. Alan will look at the county programs. We'll put an ad in Auto Trader," she gestures to Mrs. Stewart. "You're going to get the two other quotes on the gas."

I notice that as the team has moved from their original crisis mode to "empowerment" mode, the goals they are setting are tied to helping the family to become self-sufficient for the long term. Nancy is now assigning specific tasks to Mrs. Stewart to teach her how to do things for herself.

I'm impressed at how Nancy is summarizing the meeting at the end. It's too bad that Mr. Camelini isn't here to see this.

"Let's go back to the safety plan," Alan adds. "You're going to call the crisis center if you need to."

"I'm not comfortable with that, but I'll do it. It's best for everyone else," Mrs. Stewart agrees.

"Make sure you call our person on-call if you do that," Nancy adds.

"Is there anything else?" Nancy asks the group.

"I have something to say to the Stewarts," Alan says. "I feel bad about what happened with the respite worker." He turns to the rest of the group. "He just quit showing up. He needs to do some growing up. When he was there, he was great. I feel bad about that."

"It broke Kevin's heart," Mrs. Stewart responds.

"Yeah," Alan acknowledges.

"When do you want to schedule the next meeting?" Nancy asks.

"How about two months?" Mrs. Stewart offers. "That should give us time to do all this."

On the way home, I think of how the concept of power is tied up with the concept of voice. Those who have the ability to speak in a society, or as Gergen (1999) says, to "rule out all competing voices" (p. 130), are those in positions of power. In this research, I've gained a newfound appreciation for the difficulty the professionals on the teams have in equalizing their voice with the families. It's been very difficult for me to move out of the "expert researcher" role and into more of a partner role with team members.

The professionals on the team seem to experience the same tension. Families can be called "full partners" on the team, but they're still put in a subordinate position in which they're in need of help. They can voice their needs, but if the team members don't agree with what they want, they won't get it. When the family agrees with team members, their voice seems more likely to be heard than when they voice dissenting opinions. The family's voice is invited but doesn't always seem to be heard at the same level as the voice of the professionals on the team.

On the other hand, sometimes the family's voice overpowers that of the other team members. The family members, Mrs. Stewart and Kevin especially, have found effective ways of voicing resistance. When team members bring up a topic they don't want to discuss, they have an emotional out-burst that either effectively silences the rest of the team or brings them sympathy from team members. Mrs. Stewart also has been very effective in using her voice to get help. I think about how the interchange in this team meeting shows that she knows whom and how to ask for assistance. She has, in fact, received much help in response to her requests. In one sense, then, she has turned dependency into empowerment and has gained power herself by putting the professionals, Nancy and Alan especially, into a subordinate position of giving her what she asks for.

The Stewarts willingly give in to the team's power when it is in their best interest to do so. Does this, I wonder, render them less, or more, powerful? To the extent that the team is helping them in ways the team thinks is best, I think it renders them less powerful. The fact that they adhere to the "professional's" standards, labels, and practices is an indica-tion of the subjugation of power (Gergen, 1999). Yet, to the extent that they're able to manipulate the team to their own end, I think the Stewarts become more powerful.

Trying to Get Home

Today, the short and stout man on the side of the road looks like a lep-rechaun. He has a weathered face and a pointed hat. I've seen him here before; he seems to be a regular. I roll down my window to hand him a dollar.

"What's your story?" I ask. I pause momentarily, realizing that may have sounded unintentionally rude. He doesn't seem to be bothered.

"Ma'am," he says. "I'm trying to get back up home."

"Where's your home?" I ask, checking the light to make sure it's still red.

"Up north. Pennsylvania. I'm just trying to get enough money for a bus ticket."

"Oh, okay," I say.

"My girlfriend was killed a few weeks ago," he continues.

"Oh, no!" I respond. "Car accident?"

"She was hit by a car," he says. "She was drunk." He pauses. "I'll be honest, I've been hitting the sauce myself a bit lately." He wipes an eye. "It's been rough. I've got feelings, you know."

"Yeah," I say. "How awful for you! What are you planning to do when you get up to Pennsylvania?" Out of the corner of my eye, I see the light turn green. "Gotta go!

Good luck!"

"God bless you!" he responds.

CHAPTER 7

Team Voice: Constructing Voice

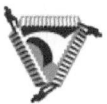

Subtle Doesn't Work

I've brought Kevin a Panthers T-shirt for his birthday. I hold my breath as he tries it on. I bought a child's size because he's so small, but then I remembered that he's 14 years old. I hope he won't be insulted at the child's shirt. To my great relief, it fits perfectly. He doesn't say anything to me, but he wears it the rest of the visit.

Sitting at Mr. and Mrs. Stewart's front table, I ask about their reactions to my reflections.

"I want to tell you some thoughts I have about the team," I begin. "I wonder if it seems that the team is being a little slow in the way they're helping make things happen."

"We think so, too," Mrs. Stewart responds quickly. Maybe too quickly, as I wonder if I just put this thought into her head or if she's been waiting for an opportunity to voice that thought.

"I'm wondering if this is just me. 'Cause I could just be being impatient," I say, trying to mediate the effect of my opinion.

"No, I'm getting a little impatient with them, too," Mrs. Stewart says. "But they have their bureaucracy."

"Lots of paperwork," Mr. Stewart adds. "That slows things down a lot, 'cause they got to have papers for this, papers for that."

Communicating Hope: An Ethnography of a Children's Mental Health Care Team by Christine S. Davis, 157–185 © 2013 Left Coast Press, Inc. All rights reserved.

"It's my belief that they want to help, but there are others in the agency that are getting in the way," Mrs. Stewart says.

"Like rules?" I attempt to clarify.

"Basically the rules of the program and how they disburse money," Mrs. Stewart explains. "The way that it was explained to me was this: The program is supposed to do whatever helps the family as long as it is not too outrageous. Helping us find a larger and better home, I don't see that that is outrageous," she adds.

"Not when you've got a home to sell," I observe. "Do you think they think it's outrageous?"

"Alan and Nancy, I don't believe they do, but there may be others who do," Mrs. Stewart responds. "Because they both said they'd like to help us."

"It's not like we're asking to move into a $300,000 mansion," says Mr. Stewart. "We showed them pictures of houses that have exactly what we want, and all the ones we've showed them have all been below $100,000 because that's what I look for. I know what we can manage and what we can't. I know what our finances are."

Mrs. Stewart adds. "Not too long ago we found one in Plant City, a 2-story, 5-bedroom, 2 bath, on 2.2 acres for $79,000, and we tried with our bank to get a loan, but the bank wouldn't go for it." My husband and I have also been in day-dreaming house-hunting mode, and I mentally wonder where the house is. Sounds perfect for us, too. I'm surprised to hear that they had talked to their bank.

"You need Alan and Nancy's help," I clarify.

"Yes, and now all of a sudden, now that we got the house almost all paid off, our bank sent us a letter saying they would give us a bank loan now. But see, we can't—there's no way we could pay off two mortgages at once. It can't be done," Mrs. Stewart answers.

I'm confused. People sell one house while buying another all the time. Did she really talk to the bank? Maybe Alan and Nancy need to explain how mortgages and real estate work.

Mr. Stewart adds, "We'd have to sell this house. Now, we did talk to *We Buy Ugly Houses*, but they offered $10,000."

I had wondered what they could get for this place.

"We paid $23,500 for this," Mrs. Stewart says. "We told them to get lost."

"Good for you," I say. "You said you had it appraised?"

"Yeah, and they said $45,000, for this house, just as it sits."

Oh, but they'd have to clean it out before they sell it, and that's the whole problem. They want to move so they don't have to clean it out. What a dilemma.

I decide to move the conversation back to reflections on the team. "What about the rest of your team? The people at the school? Peggy and Jane?"

"They hold up their end very good."

"What do they do?" I wonder.

"They help Kevin when he's in school," Mrs. Stewart responds. "When someone's trying to mess with him, they help. If he gets angry they know how to talk him down because they've seen me do it."

"What else is the team doing for you?" I ask.

Mrs. Stewart thinks for a minute. "Bus passes when we need them, and the reward money, when they all do good."

"Is that working?" I ask.

"Yes, it is working," Mrs. Stewart responds in a firm voice.

"One of the things I think they've done for you is they've provided you guys with hope. Would you agree with that?"

They nod, but make no comment, so I move on to my next observation.

"Do you remember at the last team meeting when the psychologist was there and was reading his report?" I ask.

"Yeah, I remember."

"I thought, frankly, he was being very negative," I add.

"He was being very negative," Mrs. Stewart responds.

"What did that feel like? What did you guys think about that?" I wonder.

"You want to know what I felt like?" Mrs. Stewart answers, her voice rising slightly. She gestures with her hand. "I felt like getting up and planting this right in his face. Because he don't know, he don't spend every day with Kevin."

"What did he say we were raising?" Mr. Stewart asks.

"He said we were raising a spouse abuser. That is what made me want to put my fist right in his face."

"The team usually tries to be so strengths-based. But I didn't hear this guy saying that," I continue.

"I've seen the worst side of abuse." Mrs. Stewart is still stung by the comment made, I remember, by Peggy, about her raising a spouse abuser. It's interesting that she's now attributing the comment to the school psychologist. "I was abused by my first ex-husband. He tried to murder our unborn twins while they were still in my womb. I know abuse, and if I say that I would rather take the blow than let him get it, that's not raising a child abuser. That is trying to protect, whether they like it or not. My mother, from the time I was old enough to understand, drilled into my

head that when you become a wife and mother, your duty, your responsibility of love is to protect all, not just one, but all. If they can't get that
through their heads, that is their problem. I'm going to do whatever I
think is necessary and right to protect my family, even if it means getting
hit by Kevin. Whether they like it or not."

"Do you think the team understands that?" I wonder, as I notice what
a strong belief this is for her.

"No, I don't believe they do!" Mrs. Stewart says forcefully. "Because
I tried to explain it to them and they kept cutting me off. They want to
help, and I appreciate them wanting to help. But they got to understand
the type of family I was raised up in where the mother is the chief protec-
tor of all, because that is the way it was meant to be. Even in the animals,
the female protects her children." What an interesting point of view, I
think.

"What do you wish the team would do differently?" I ask.

"Not be so prejudging," Mrs. Stewart responds. "Listen to us. The
type of lifestyle that they grew up with is different than ours. They grew
up in families that probably had a lot more money. A lot less stress and
strain."

"I think that, too," I confess. "What makes you think that?"

"It's just the expression on their faces that I see, the disbelief," she
says. "The disgust. Like when I talked about taking the hits instead of letting Kevin hit him or Karla or Gary. It was the disgust that I saw on their
face that made me very upset. Why should I stand by and let anyone get
hit when I can intercept it and maybe even stop it before the blow even
lands? That's basically what I was trying to get through to them. When
I put myself in between it's not because I want to get hit. It's because I
think that I'm fast enough that I can prevent the blow from even landing.
Which is something that they don't want to get through their heads. I'm
very quick."

"They're really alarmed about the thought of your getting hit," I
observe.

She shrugs. "I've been hit so many times, it would hurt, but other than
that it wouldn't bother me. I got used to it. I don't like the pain, but I can
deal with it. That's what I tried to tell them."

"Do you think it's because their culture is very different from yours?"

Mrs. Stewart agrees. "Their culture is very different. We've been trying
to get through to Kevin, that you never hit somebody unless they hit you
first. Like my father said, never start a fight, but if somebody else starts it,
you better finish it. Never walk away. I've finished more than my share."

"If the team understood that more and understood the way your culture is, what would they be doing differently?" I ask.

"They probably would be more understanding," Mr. Stewart responds. "When we grew up, we didn't have money to go to Busch Gardens or Disney World regularly. A lot of times we ate beans and rice for supper and that was it."

I nod.

Mrs. Stewart adds. "When I was growing up, our recreation was limited to going to the movies."

"What would the team be doing differently then, if they understood all that?" I ask.

"They'd be less critical and they'd be trying to assist us a lot more than what they've been doing," she says.

I continue. "What would you like them to assist you with?"

"Getting a new house," she says. "That is our number one priority. After that, Disney World for Christmas one year, that's off in the future, but right now our main priority is getting a bigger house and bigger property."

"How would you describe the way the team communicates with you?" I ask.

"With Alan and Nancy it's okay, but with other members of the team, it's not that good," Mrs. Stewart responds.

"Can you give me an example?" I ask.

She says, "I'll use that school psychologist for instance. The other one, Peggy—she's the one that actually said that we were raising a spouse abuser." So she did remember who said that. I thought she'd been acting in meetings toward Peggy as if she was still hurt by the comment.

"Why do you think she said that?" I wonder.

Mrs. Stewart frowns. "Because she doesn't understand what my basic goal is, to keep Kevin safe but to keep him from hurting anyone else. If I have to physically intervene and restrain him in some way, even if I get hit in the process of restraining him, then it's better for him," she says.

"So she just doesn't get it," I clarify.

"No, she doesn't get it. When I tried to explain to her . . ." her voice trails off.

"What would you like to say to her?" I ask.

"I would like to tell her, look, the type of culture you were raised in and the type of culture I was raised in are entirely different. They're miles apart. They're even thousands of dollars apart. You were probably an only child. Your parents had money all the time to do whatever ya'll wanted to do, to go wherever ya'll wanted to go. My family didn't."

I've had a feeling that Mrs. Stewart and Peggy were holding back saying things to each other. "Why have you not said that to her? Do you think you could say it to her?"

"Yeah, but I don't want to offend her. People that come from money sometimes get offended." Interesting. I never would have said that Peggy comes from money.

"She's a nice lady." I feel compelled to defend her, because I really believe that Peggy is being unfairly singled out by Mrs. Stewart.

"I know she is," Mrs. Stewart responds. "I like her."

"That's why I'm asking you about this," I continue, "because I really do think that everyone on the team has good intentions, but clearly there's something . . ."

"I like her," Mrs. Stewart interrupts. "But she needs to understand the type. If you look at things logically, the families that he and I came from are considered low class. Very low income. In other words, to put it bluntly, poor. We still are. She does not see the stresses and strains that puts on us. We don't even have the $25 to pay our friends for the scooter they bought for him. There's a big difference between a family that dips into savings when something like that happens and a family that doesn't eat when something like that happens."

I nod. She is so perceptive. There was a time in my life when I was the latter. Now, I'm thankful for having the savings to dip into.

She continues. "The team's helped us get the paint for the outside of the house. I know the porch still needs painting. We just haven't got around to it. But we've got the outside painted, and that's what code enforcement wanted."

"So they helped you with that," I say.

"They helped us get the materials to build a new bathroom," Mr. Stewart remembers.

"That's right," I say.

"They were surprised that we could take what they gave us and go to Home Depot, and find bargains because we know where to look. Paint that is out of stock, $15 for 5 gallons, and we found two of them. We got the rollers, the paint brushes, the sealers, everything we needed, for $200. We had $17 of it left over," Mr. Stewart says, bragging a bit.

"They should hire you to help other families learn how to save money," I say, meaning it.

"Lowe's is a rip-off. Don't go to Lowe's," he responds.

"My interest is in studying the way the team communicates with you, and whether or not it helps you," I say.

"Well," Mrs. Stewart responds, "if they understood us more, where we grew up, and the times back when we were growing up. There was gas rationing—we all lived through that. Ten gallons a week is all they were letting people get. We couldn't hardly go anywhere unless we scrounged up extra money. That's how I learned about aluminum cans. That's how we got our extra money for gas so we could go places like the movies."

Mr. Stewart nods. "They got to realize that our family here, if something happens, if the van breaks down, or like the gas company happened, it's devastating to us."

"Yeah," I acknowledge with a nod, then continue with my questions. "So, what's the best interaction you've had with your team? What's the best time you've been together with them?"

"I think the first meeting we ever had was the best time," she responds. I'm a little surprised. I remember that my first impression was that the team wasn't doing much for the family at first. "After that, they got where they were talking more clinical things as opposed to the actual human facts of the entire situation." Interesting, I think.

"Tell me about that first time that was best. What made it the best?" I wonder.

"They listened to us. They were trying to understand what we go through, and that was the first time that Kevin actually acted up and they saw how I dealt with it, and at the time they were very impressed by it. Now, I don't think that they are; they're starting to see things through a microscope instead of with their own eyes. If they keep doing it, it's not going to work."

"What's the worst interaction you've had?" I ask.

"The last meeting that we had when they accused us of raising a spouse abuser. That was the worst one right there," Mrs. Stewart remembers. I notice she remembers that happened in the last team meeting. There have been many team meetings and interactions since then.

"Do you feel like you're an equal member of the team? Equal to everyone else?" I ask.

"Yeah," Mrs. Stewart responds.

"What do they do to make you feel like you're equal to the rest of the team?" I ask.

"Sometimes they listen to me," Mr. Stewart says.

"He said sometimes," Mrs. Stewart points out. "That's the thing with us. They don't listen all the time and they should. They need to listen to what is actually pertinent to the whole family group, not just what's pertinent to Kevin."

"So you think that they concentrate more on Kevin than the whole family," I observe.

"In a way, yes. You have to look at it as a whole. We're individuals but we're still a group. We are one solid family unit. You can't just look at only one individual instead of the whole and say that everything being done is right. 'Cause we're more than just the sum of our parts. That's what they need to understand. We are a circle. That's just the way it is. We do what benefits all of us, that's why it goes in a circle, what is best for all of us is best for one."

I'm fascinated. It's as if she's sat in on one of my lectures on systems theory. She seems to have a wealth of knowledge that she holds back. I wonder what else is in her mind that we don't know about.

She continues, "Because one family member affects the other."

"They don't always understand that," I clarify.

"No. What they need to understand is we are a whole. We are a family," Mrs. Stewart responds. "See, when Kevin acts up . . ."

"It affects all of us," Mr. Stewart finishes her sentence.

"How would they treat you differently if they understood that?" I ask.

"They probably would have a lot more respect and understanding and consideration for us. Mostly Peggy is the one that needs to understand where we come from," Mrs. Stewart says. She's really holding a grudge against Peggy for her comment, I think to myself.

"She doesn't understand me," Kevin says from the living room couch in front of the television. It's the first comment he's made since I got here. I hadn't realized he was listening to us.

"What does she do to make you think that?" I ask.

"She acts like she doesn't even hear me," he answers. "Like she don't even care." I wonder if that's true or if the whole family is demonizing her for her comment.

I continue. "If you were me, writing research about how the team communicates and whether or not it helps you, what should I know? What should you make sure that I know when I'm writing?"

Mrs. Stewart responds. "If it was me, how to communicate better, listen more to what we say. Try to be more understanding, more considerate, more compassionate about the situations that we grew up in and the situations that we're in now. See, Kevin is a unique person. They all are unique, each with their different strengths and weaknesses. Our biggest strength is learning how to deal with their uniqueness. If the team understood more about us as people instead of just parents of an ADHD child, they would understand us better."

"If they knew you as individuals," I observe.

"Yes. They see us as a group, but they don't see us as the individual entities that we are. We have different ideas about things than they do," she responds, now doing a textbook job of describing the developmental view of interpersonal communication.

I want to go back to their resentment of Peggy for expressing what I saw as obvious concern for the whole family. I feel sorry for Peggy for their anger toward her, yet I also understand how they could be angry. I'd probably feel exactly the same way if someone said that to me, especially in front of other people. Yet, I know Peggy meant well and has done quite a bit of good for the family.

I temper my question because I'm afraid that it will make Mrs. Stewart angry. "Let me ask you, 'cause this is a question I don't have the answer to, and I don't know if anybody does. If a person thinks that something would be harmful, like a child hitting you or something, is it more important for them to be respectful of your culture, or is it more important for them to express what they think is right?" I hope she doesn't take offense at my question.

"They should find an even balance between their clinical knowledge and the way things really are with the family they're helping," she responds.

"You know your family better than them," Mr. Stewart adds.

"See, to be able to help properly, they've got to have an adequate balance of both," Mrs. Stewart continues. "They've got to have the clinical knowledge, but they also have to have a personal understanding of the family's emotional, physical, financial, and cultural situation to be able to do what they want to do properly." What a great answer, I think.

She continues with the specific example. "We don't want Kevin to do what he does, so it's not that anybody thinks what he's doing is okay. It's just the way you're looking at it. It's not okay, but if I take a blow because I'm trying to intercept him before he can hit somebody—while it is not acceptable—I can live with whatever pain the blow causes."

I think that underneath her pain and anger is the desire to be seen as a person who makes logical choices in a bad situation. I respond, "Sure, I understand. I understand what you're saying."

I think of another question I really wonder about. "What do you think it felt like to Kevin to have that psychologist talk about the test results like that?"

Mrs. Stewart frowns. "It made him very sad. When he came home, he did something that I very rarely ever see him do. He was crying. When he got off the bus, he was crying already. He went straight to his room and he didn't talk to nobody. He didn't even want to eat supper. He didn't want to do anything."

The emotion in her answer almost seems melodramatic. I wonder if that's true or if she's performing what she thinks I want to hear. "I think it upset the whole team," I reflect. "Nancy tried to turn it around."

"I know she did, so did I," Mrs. Stewart responds. "But if he would have kept on opening his mouth, I'd have shut it. To put it bluntly, he thinks he knows more than God and everyone else. He knows absolutely nothing about us or Kevin."

I nod. "I think he forgot that there were people behind those numbers."

"He's got to see us as humans first, and then a clinical study next," Mrs. Stewart says. "The human factor always has to come first." I couldn't have said it better myself, I think.

She continues. "We all have different ideas and different belief systems about things as they are. See, clinical psychologists, you excluded . . ."

I interrupt her. "I'm not one—that ain't my area!" I say with emphasis.

"But you ultimately want to be one," she says.

I clarify, "No. I'm a communication scholar. That's my area."

She's insistent. "Eventually you may want to go into clinical psychology."

I'm insistent back. "What I want to do is teach them how to communicate."

Finally, she seems to understand and gives me advice. "What they need to understand is that all people are different. People come from different cultures, races, financial situations, religious belief systems. When you add together their belief system—whether it's religious or cultural or both—and their financial situation, you get a very complex family unit. That's what they need to understand and learn about. If those people could live with us and see us as we really are, see the day-to-day stresses and strains that we go through, they would be a lot more inclined to ignore the numbers. They got this list of numbers, and they say all these people have to fit in with this list of numbers, and we don't fit. We are outside of those numbers. I'll put it like this: We are something they've never been exposed to. We are a family that puts the family first, not the individual but the whole group." She is speaking passionately. Again I think that she's been holding back an awful lot of knowledge and insight.

I think for a minute. "Could I repeat this at the focus group and get their reaction to it?"

She doesn't hesitate. "Sure. Be my guest. You can use whatever I said."

I continue. "Do you want me just to say it, or do you want me to say that you said it? 'Cause I don't want to embarrass you or put you in an awkward situation."

"It wouldn't embarrass me and it wouldn't put me in an awkward situation."

"I just want to make sure," I say.

"I'm going to leave that to your best judgment. Whatever you think is best, the way you want to put it is fine with me." Me in the expert role again!

I have one last question. "Talk about me and what I'm doing with the group."

"You've been very helpful, because some of the ideas I've expressed to you, I don't know the exact way to say it. They'll understand you." She sees me as her opportunity to have voice in the team.

Is that an appropriate role for me? "I'm afraid that sometimes I interfere a little too much."

"I don't believe so," she says. "You don't interfere."

I continue. "Sometimes there are just some things I don't think they're hearing," I confess.

She agrees. "They're not hearing. Tell them!"

"I'm trying to be subtle about it, but I have," I say.

She leans forward. "Can I give you a bit of advice?"

I nod. "Yes. Absolutely."

"Forget subtle. Forget subtle."

I stifle a laugh as I remember who I'm talking to. Mrs. Stewart is definitely not into subtle. She continues. "Subtle doesn't work."

Subtle doesn't get you voice, I think.

People like the Stewarts who are marginalized don't expect to be given voice; they're socialized to believe that their voice won't be heard (Farmer, 2003). The Stewarts are used to being muted by society—disconfirmed and discounted. In the past, their requests for help have not been responded to. To be given voice is to be publicly confirmed, acknowledged, and heard. Voice asserts the interconnectedness of people in a discourse community (Watts, 2001). I think about how much of this story is one of voice and muting. Mrs. Stewart and Kevin are struggling to be heard. Team members struggle to be heard by the Stewarts. Nancy struggles to be heard by the team. Team members' presence and absence are felt throughout the process, as their voice is either silent or present. Mrs. Stewart and Kevin try to force their voice through their emotionality. They seem to understand intuitively that emotional intensity of voice enhances empathy from others (Watts, 2001).

"What would you like me to tell them for you?" I ask.

"For me? Tell them to shut their mouth and open up their ears, their hearts and their mind. They're too much lip service. If they really want to understand us, they need to look at us, not through the eyes of clinical numbers or established procedures. They've got to start looking at us with their hearts and the emotional part of their mind. Put the clinical stuff in the file cabinet, lock it up, and leave it there. They forget that they're people, too."

I think ahead to my research analysis. "So here's how I would put it. I would say that they need to connect with you at the human level."

"Exactly. They forget they're people. There's the title: teacher, clinical psychologist, psychiatrist, psychoanalyst," she says.

"Parent," I add. "All those titles get in the way, don't they?"

"Parent. *Parent* is not so much a title as it is a description of what we do. Like the word *family*. That's not a title. That is a description of the whole. Which is what they can't get past. There's all these titles, and they can't get past those titles. Until they can, they're not going to be able to see us as we are. That's what they need to do, to see us as we actually are."

What a great comment to end the conversation with, I think, as Kevin walks me to my car. He makes a big show of opening my car door for me.

"Thank you, sir!" I say. "What great manners you have!"

The drive home is swift, as thoughts swirl around in my brain. The contrast of the Stewart's home with the culture around them is striking, and it sets them up as "different," on the margins of society. They're poorer than average. Their house is smaller than most. It's dirtier than is acceptable in our society. It's in more disrepair than is allowed. It's more cluttered than is appropriate. Kevin's behavior is more emotional than normal. His test scores are less than average. They're more needy than most. Their children have no sense of place—no space to call their own, no space to be alone and be themselves. In a society that values individualism and space, this is a huge deviancy.

Our society tends to divide people into "us " and "others"—that's how we construct a sense of identity, morality, and community, by separating those who can produce from those who need help (Gergen, 1999; Oliver, 1990). Unfortunately, as we do that, we tend to avoid "the others," oversimplify who they are, and find fault with their behaviors. In fact, disability is one way that we dominate others, by moving people with problems away from us—to "special" schools, classrooms, or neighborhoods, as we insure society's unfamiliarity with them and increase the likelihood of seeing them as "others" (Oliver, 1990; Zola, 2004). We deal with people with more needs and problems than the rest of us by marginalizing them, stigmatizing them, medicalizing them, and by finding fault with them. We tend to blame people who are poor for their poverty, disabled for their disability, and mentally ill for their behavior and ignore the influence of culture and society on their situation (Farmer, 2003; Oliver, 1990; Watts, 2001).

As Haley (1963) points out: "To say that a person with a symptom is behaving in a way that is out of the ordinary implies that there is an ordinary way to behave" (p. 6). When we see normal problems of daily life as "illnesses," we tend to disempower people's own abilities to solve their own problems and blame people who have these problems (Gergen, 1999). When we situate problems in the individual, we ignore the systemic nature of circumstances and situations (Gergen, 1999). What if it isn't the person who is broken but the situation? Or the system? Or society?

Yet, despite our divisions and differences, I think about how relationships are developing on the team. Through Warren's efforts to show the kids in Kevin's classroom that Kevin is like them, and Alan's efforts to show the team that Mrs. Stewart is like them (reacting to circumstances the same way any of us would), relationships are beginning to develop.

I think about the Stewarts' advice in this interview. What are the takeaways? Listen to us. Understand us. Relate to us, to where we're from and how we were raised. Treat us like people, not problems. Look at our family unit. Show us respect. Get to know us as unique individuals not just as stereotypes of our problems or situations. Trust our own expertise and knowledge of our situation. Look at us at the level at which we're the same as you—human beings with strengths and challenges, knowledge, and resources. Understand that how we do what we do is a logical response to an undesirable situation.

It's Crazy Out There

Today, the leprechaun guy is at my exit again. "Still, here, I see!" I say, as I hand him a dollar.

"Yeah, I still need a few more dollars to get home," he says.

I nod.

"It's crazy out here!" he observes. "I've been sleeping in the woods, and there's some crazy people out here!"

"It's probably not too safe, either," I say with concern. I wave as the light changes. "Stay safe and have a good trip!"

"Thank you, darling!" he responds. I'd normally be insulted at being called "darling" by a stranger, but today, it sounds nice.

Feeling More Hopeful

Two weeks later, I have a chance to discuss my ideas about the research with Nancy and Alan. We're at Jason's Deli again. I eat here at least once a week. I munch on salad as we talk and as I shuffle through notes in front of me.

"One of the things that I'm trying to do with this research," I explain, "is to not be the expert, imposing my opinion on the rest of the team. I want this to be a partnership between me and the team. One of the things I'm discovering is how hard it is not to play the expert role. I wonder if it's hard for you and all the other professionals on the team to have the family be a real true partner on the team."

Nancy answers first. "The more frequently the team meets, the better it is to have them be viewed as a full partner. It's much better that there is a team, because otherwise they're asking me for things. This way, I can say wait for the team to decide instead of being the gatekeeper. I also think the team realizes their partnership more when they meet regularly."

Alan nods. "We've talked about this before. You have a situation of power, no matter what. If you're just talking about us being case managers, I don't even think about it anymore, being the professional versus the family, because we just do what we need to do to get things better."

"But isn't the power differential still there, even if you don't think about it?" I protest.

"To complicate matters," Nancy adds, "the financial assistance fund puts them in a subservient role since they have to ask for it, and it's the state's money. We have to make decisions that are not just about adhering to the family's choice. A good example is the situation with the gas. I can't as an administrator just hand them the money because she wanted to go specifically to another, more expensive, company because she was mad at the first company. By statutes, I had to say no, and that was a power decision. But I don't know that power necessarily needs to be looked at as something that is either inherently positive or negative. It's how you use it."

"How about the other professionals on the team?"

"That depends. As far as the regular team members, I don't know that I've been aware of any abuse of power or anything like that. The school psychologist definitely came over as the big expert, talking about a lot of negative things," Alan says.

"He didn't really understand our team," Nancy adds. "He was just invited that day as a guest."

"I don't think it was his fault," Alan responds, "but he came over powerfully and very negatively. I don't think it was his intention to do that, but at the same time I don't think he saw that family with the level of respect that the team members that know them do."

I nod. "I felt that he dehumanized them. Would you agree with that?"

Alan smiles. "I think that's what I just said."

"I've been noticing how the family, especially Kevin, seems to be doing better, and I wonder why you think that is," I ask.

Nancy sits forward. "I've thought a lot about this. We've given them more structure. The family financially isn't able to go a lot of places, and with the behavioral rewards, now they have something to look forward to every week. On Monday, they're already looking forward to what they're going to do on Saturday, and so they have a hope of things getting better."

Hope. Interesting.

She continues. "Also, they have frequent contact with me. So if there's a problem, they don't have a feeling that nobody wants to listen to us, that there's nowhere to go with this."

"What's that like?" I ask, feeling frustrated that she hasn't let me know about interactions to observe for this research.

"This summer, I've been coming out to their house. I always call and tell them when I'm coming. By the time I get there, they're watching for the car. I can't even get out of the car, 'cause they're all at my door. All the kids, both the parents. Everybody wants to talk, and they all talk about their week. Everyone seems to be very open."

"In terms of their behavior?" I clarify.

She responds. "What they've been doing, and their behavior. They're very open to talking about what's going on with the behavior contract."

I can't resist a subtle hint. "I ought to go with you one time and watch that." She doesn't respond, and I change the subject. "The main question for my research is to look at what this team is constructing for themselves and the family, and I think one of the things that the team is constructing is hope."

They nod and I continue. "Alan, you and I have talked several times about this. One way you all are doing this is by changing your focus from the past and the present into the future. The past is problem-saturated. The present ain't so hot either, right? But when you focus them on the future, whether it's for the weekend, or next year when they'll have a bigger house, I think that's being hopeful. Could you all comment on that?"

Nancy nods. "Yeah, I do agree. The other thing I think is that Mrs. Stewart doesn't see the team as impersonal. They may be straightforward with her about their opinion, but she doesn't doubt that they care about them and her children. That's created a different dynamic, 'cause she's not feeling like it's an 'us versus them' thing."

Alan interjects. "I think it's much more complicated than just hope. I agree that, in general, what we do and hope for is to improve and nurture. I also think that with this family, there's not an adversarial relationship within the team. We may have disagreements, but I don't see it being adversarial. Mrs. Stewart was very defensive at first, and everyone has done a nice job of getting to the point where it's a group of people that are in a non-adversarial relationship."

Hmmm. I'm not entirely sure that's true after my interview with the family. How interesting different points of view are.

"What has caused that, do you think?" I wonder.

"Everybody has worked towards that, in their different roles," Alan responds. "The school system people on the team have demonstrated they do care about the kid and they want the best for his education. They've worked real hard despite bureaucratic frustrations to have an evaluation done, and they've supported change and movement as far as his education. So it's talking and supporting, but also doing. I think the family has moved in a direction of being much more willing to listen. They've improved. They've chosen to develop a level of trust and a level of closeness as far as the relationship is concerned."

"In the family?" I attempt to clarify.

"Within the team," he says. "We've tried as much as we can to follow our values and what our job description is. We've tried real hard not to work in an adversarial manner, even though we've had some disagreements and we've had to say no. I think that's nice because we've been able to do that, and they've been pissed at us, and we've been pissed at them, but I don't believe it's adversarial. The other thing is, if you're going to act as change agents, and we are, you can't deal with the past other than just for information. You have to take a proactive approach and look at changing the future. I don't think it's just about hope, although that's in there, but without some of those other things, I think, quite frankly, hope can be hollow. We're not working just for hollow hope here."

Well said, I think. But, I think to myself, isn't that what hope is all about, looking to the future proactively?

"I've recently read some research that says there's a lot of different dimensions to hope." I read from the notes I have in front of me. "There's realistic hope, false hope, hope as acceptance, no hope, hope in faith, living in hope, having something to hope for, hope in the future, hope as part of a relationship, and hope that's a type of resilience [Hammer, Mogensen, & Hall, 2009; Soundy et al., 2010]. Regardless of the approach to hope, I do think there's a fine line between real hope and false hope. How do you walk that line and not give families false hope?" I ask.

"Being honest," Alan responds. "I think it's a roller coaster that you manage differently as time goes on, but probably a really good example is this house."

"Yeah."

Alan continues. "I was gung-ho on the house before June, we were going to work hard to get this done, because I was feeling empathy, sympathy, and a desire to see this family in a different place. We now have information from people that we consider experts that has brought me down to, I think, to a much more real, realistic approach to this house thing."

Yeah, what about that house? "What are you going to do about the house?"

"The house plan is not going to work," Alan responds. Oops. "I frankly think I got carried away with the idea, and I built up false hope for them. I feel bad about that." Double oops. I guess I did, too.

Alan continues. "I think that's part of the thing with the team. I think sometimes the team forms its own opinion of things, and it changes as time goes on. We have information now that we didn't have previously, and now we've got to be honest and talk about that and see where they want to go, where the team wants to go from there. I know Mrs. Stewart is really, really intent on getting a new house. But the way the real estate system is, if they don't have any credit, they can't get credit. They have a fixed income that's not looked on by any lender as being a desired type of income. Plus, their house will be impossible to sell, according to the realtor."

That's not fair! I think to myself. I can't think of more steady income than federal disability income! Their current house is almost paid off! Doesn't that count for something? I focus my attention back on Alan.

"I think we may have all had some false hope together, and now we've got to get ourselves realistic," he says.

"Does that make hope bad, then, if it will cause them to feel let down?" I ask.

"I don't think so," he responds. "They can hope for other things, too. I think hope has to be realistic. We can all hope we're going to win the lottery this week, but sometimes it may have to be adjusted a bit to what's realistically possible."

Nancy jumps into the conversation. "I do think that just having a team is a big part of it. For example, the first time I met Kevin was at a meeting at his former school, and at that first meeting the agenda was to get him out of that school. That was all they wanted to do at that meeting— get him out of that school, and they did. They didn't even continue the meeting; it was a done thing. Now the family knows that while we may not always have the answers they want to hear, we won't ignore them. We won't be unresponsive. We're there, and that means a lot."

Unconditional positive regard, perhaps, I think. I change the subject. "I've seen what I think are a series of tensions that I think are building toward hope. There's this tension between deviance and being normal."

Alan straightens his back. "Define deviance."

Whoops. Jargon. "Being different, but different in a bad way. In our society, people are considered deviant socially in a lot of ways—mentally ill people in our society are deviant. People who are in prison are deviant."

Alan shakes his head. "I don't see them as being deviant. Not in the terms that you're using, because you're using it in a bad way. Now, in a psychological sense I do see pathology. But I don't see that as bad. A person who's depressed, they're pathological, but that's not bad. I do have a lot of empathy for them, but I also don't see them as normal."

"Tell me more about that," I say.

"Kevin has all kinds of learning disabilities," Alan says. "He has neurological problems, and he has some very different, oppositional defiance types of things that would lead up to a diagnosis. He's in the most severe academic placement you can be in, in our county. I don't consider that normal. But yet he's a really neat kid whom I like a lot. I want the best for him and would like a part in being able to help him. I actually don't see him negatively. Does that make sense?"

"Yeah, it makes perfect sense," I respond.

Nancy sits thoughtfully for a minute. "When I look at the family in general, they do have a lot of issues. Economically, they're probably struggling as hard or harder than most families, and neither one of the parents is employed, which is unusual in our culture. One has a chronic physical illness, one has mental health issues. I guess I'm having a problem with the idea of deviant. Now, if you're looking at some sort of bell curve, they're not in the middle."

"No," I agree.

"Maybe outliers," she continues. "The word deviant has a real different connotation to both of us than the thought that we have about the families we work with. We may just be reacting to that word," she says.

I respond. "I'm glad you are, and I am using a harsh word on purpose, because I think that your training has led you to have a great deal of empathy. I think you can have empathy for them and see them as worthwhile people worthy of admiration, in spite of recognizing they're not what you'd call normal. I think that's the other side of the coin. But this is not a family that a lot of people in our culture would be comfortable sitting down at the dinner table with."

Alan disagrees. "They're a lot like my relatives down in Riverview. Actually, they're exactly like my relatives down in Riverview."

I'm skeptical. "Really?"

"Yeah. Good old boy. They go to their drag races. Mr. Stewart's dad used to race cars there. When I was a kid, my oldest sister Harriet, who lived in Riverview, used to take me down there all the time. I probably saw his father race, but I don't remember his name. They're just like my own relatives."

I nod. "We've talked a few times about how they remind me of a family that would be in Appalachia a generation ago. They're deviant, or different, because they seem to be in the wrong place at the wrong time to fit in with the rest of society."

Nancy thinks for a minute and says, "I'm not real comfortable with that word either. But, I think of the bell curve. They clearly are not in the middle. They step back in history in the way they look at the world. Their world is full of technology; they've got videotapes and TV. Yet, they don't seem to have really caught up to where we are in their view of the world."

I agree. "Part of it I think is cultural competence. I was chatting with the family about culture. I think this family is of a different culture from most everybody else. I think a lot of their situation is about a lack of socialization into the dominant culture. We could be really culturally competent and say this is the way they are, let's just work within their culture. But what does that mean for the kids who are going to have to live in the dominant culture that doesn't understand them?"

Nancy nods. "It's just like taking someone from the movie *Coal Miner's Daughter* and plunking them down in the middle of the city."

"That's exactly right. Unfortunately, there are not a whole lot of places they can go to fit in." I continue with my thought, "So, given that cultural competence is one of your philosophies, how do you reconcile that? Being respectful of their culture while realizing that if you don't somehow try to change them out of their culture, the kids may not be able to function. The parents may not be able to function for the rest of their lives."

Alan responds. "I don't believe that practicing cultural competency locks you in to stepping away from working with the family to better themselves. Or to adapt to being able to be functional."

"What if they really don't want to?" I ask.

"We can't make them," Nancy responds.

"What if they think they're functional the way they are?" I add. "'Cause they're functioning!"

Alan says, "Yeah, but they want better for their kids. Both Mom and Dad want their kids to finish school. They want their daughter not to get knocked up until she's married. They see they need to do something better. They have a vested interest to see that those three kids are in school, because they see school as a way out of where they are. I get back to the evolutionary stuff. Human beings adapt or die. We can respect the heck out of the Neanderthals and their culture and have great fascination over it, but they're dead. They died 'cause they couldn't adapt. These three kids have to adapt and learn and cope with things that they may not find at home, and I think that's partially our responsibility to help them do that, but I don't see that as not being culturally competent."

Nancy agrees. "Yeah, I don't either. I think all the team is very respectful of their family's culture, their family's traditions. But I don't have any problem discussing with them changing their parenting, for instance. I don't ever criticize where they are culturally, but I also don't shy away when I think it's appropriate. They don't live on a farm on 50 acres where they can grow all they eat and make their own soap. They don't. They live in the middle of the city, so you have to have certain kinds of survival skills."

I decide to move on to a question about my next reflection. "What's the role of trust in this team?"

Nancy responds. "I think it's really fundamental. I think that it's actually probably the foundation of the team, because if you don't have trust about what you share, or trust that what you reveal will be treated respectfully, you'll reveal a lot less and you'll deal with the issues a lot less. That's part of watching a relationship grow, it's something that you do your best to always do what you say you're going to do. Call back, answer people. That doesn't mean that you're going to say yes or agree with everything, but it means to be respectful, to always be available. The key is when they reveal something, that they're not criticized, even if it's something that the team doesn't agree with, tell them why and listen."

"Trust is this roller coaster played out over time with ever-increasing levels," Alan says philosophically. "Trust is a very critical and important thing. They needed to be able to trust other folks, and I think that has a lot to do with hope, 'cause I think you have to trust people to have hope. They can't succeed by themselves. With this family it's been a roller coaster, back and forth, up and down. Does that make sense?"

"It makes perfect sense to me," I respond. "What about boundaries?"

Nancy answers. "I have probably right now the most contact with the family of any of the team members, so I have more of a balancing act. They want certain things that can't happen, so the mom seems pretty excitable, emotional sometimes. I guess there's at least enough trust that I'll always get back to her and I'll listen to her. She can escalate pretty quickly, especially if she has her mind set on something." She pauses. "What was your question?"

"Boundaries."

"Boundaries. With this family, I have to keep boundaries, because if I didn't, we'd be all over the place. I don't have a problem with it, but she calls me on weekends. But we keep the boundaries, and it really hasn't been a problem. I don't think it has been for any of the team members."

I continue. "Talk to me about vulnerability."

Nancy responds. "With Mrs. Stewart, her emotion can change real quickly. When she wants something and she doesn't get it, you can see her emotionality. I think they are very vulnerable. In our community, they're vulnerable to people's impression to not getting heard or listened to respectfully sometimes, or people making up their minds too quickly in thinking they understand a situation that's really very complex. It felt that way when the psychologist boiled everything down to testing. They are vulnerable in a lot of ways. They're trying to hold their family together the best way that they know how, and they have a lot of vulnerabilities. Economically, healthwise, mental healthwise."

Alan adds, "They're vulnerable enough to where I think we could very easily classify them as at-risk on quite a few dimensions. They're at risk for losing their house because it isn't up to code. They're at risk for being in the hospital and dying because of medical conditions. They're at risk for doing a few things that would put their kids in foster care. So yeah, I see this family as very, very vulnerable. But at the same time, they are also a very strong family in a lot of different areas. Remember Peggy and that thing with the Baker Act stuff and how Mom went ballistic. After that, Peggy was very clear about the fact that she was off base with that. She said she was glad that we looked at it in a different way, and she really backed off from her position, and I think that was a vulnerability."

Interesting. Peggy mentioned to me in our interview that she regretted saying it the way she said it, but I don't remember her expressing regret in any team meeting. I know Mrs. Stewart didn't hear that from her.

Nancy adds, "At that team meeting, Warren talked openly about his own background growing up in foster care. He talked about the system and what it can be like to need things that you don't know how to get from the school. He tried to explain how Kevin was a lot more vulnerable than he looked like he was to the community, the school, whatever. That he was actually very different and didn't know how to relate to other kids. Warren shared that vulnerability that he had had growing up and that gave him a lot of empathy for the family."

"Talk to me about empowerment and disempowerment," I ask.

"The whole idea of the team approach," Nancy responds, "is to have a family feel listened to and heard, and think people really do care what they say. If it's something that we can help with we'll say yes. There's actually a lot that we can help with, probably more than the family realized. I do think that they think they have a lot of input in their plan. It's not just a bunch of people sitting around saying 'okay now, do this.' I think feelings of empowerment have increased in team members, too. Even the teacher said he doesn't feel so alone."

I look down at the papers in front of me. "I've got some notes here from an article," I say, "that says that you empower team members by helping them to identify with the team by clarifying roles and sharing ideas. You also empower team members by giving them autonomy—making them responsible for their results. Helping them take advantage of the team approach, focusing on results, and encouraging one another, is also empowering" [Müllern & Nordin, 2012]. I pause as Nancy nods.

"But here's something else I'm struggling with—how about the issue of helping and not helping?" I ask.

Nancy responds. "Anything to do with safety, with helping them be the best they can be, helping them fulfill whatever their potential is, that to me is really helping. They can tell you what they want help with. We can give them a bunch of temporary stuff, and I try to be respectful, but I say, 'okay, you want more? You may have to go to work even though maybe it's not what you want. If you want more income, you may have to change what your functioning is.' Like the bus pass issue. This is a microcosm of the question, because we can give them bus passes until one day the bus passes will go away. If we can work on how the family is going to get from place A to B, and get their appointments solved, that's helping. Helping them and creating dependency on something that's going to go away is not helping."

That's exactly what the literature says, too, I think. But, there's just something about it in practice that doesn't feel right. Does the family know why sometimes they're helped and sometimes they're not? If getting them a bigger house would allow Mrs. Stewart to start a home crafts business, isn't that empowering helping?

Alan's comment to Nancy breaks into my thoughts. "That gets to what I think is the fine job that you're doing pushing Mom into getting her driver's license. I think that's a step toward more independence."

"Or income to keep getting her own bus passes, if she's not getting her driver's license. Long-range thinking," Nancy adds.

Alan sits forward. "I think really pushing that stuff is a good thing. Interestingly enough though, we're using our power. Are we using our power in the way the family wants us to? Not at all. But we're bound by our ethics to do no harm and to not create dependency, so yes. We struggle with this, do we help to form dependencies or do we help form independence? I don't know. With this specific family, I sometimes think I do a good job. I sometimes think I don't do a good job. I don't think I did a good job with this thing with the house. I should have kept my mouth shut a lot more with this family about the house than I did."

Maybe I should have, too, I think guiltily.

Alan continues. "Or I should have really modulated my feelings of hope, which I believe were even nonverbally communicated, until I got more data. I don't think that was a good thing for me to have done. Now I won't do it again, so I learned my lesson."

How can you give up so fast on this idea? I think to myself. Just because Plan A doesn't work, doesn't mean there's not a Plan B? Is giving the family hope a bad thing? Or am I just feeling defensive here since my enthusiasm and prodding got Alan excited about the idea in the first place?

I tune back in to what Alan's saying. "But that probably is not going to end up helping this family, it's going to make them more discouraged for a while, and they'll have to adapt. One of the things I realize is that it's important for me to be aware of when I should allow somebody to be in pain. Pain can bring about change. I need to be really self-conscious of when I'm doing something just to relieve pain or discomfort, without evaluating that distress and pain enough to make a much more cautious decision about whether I should intervene, or let it go. Because if you're not in pain, no change." Very interesting. So, letting people stay in pain might actually be helping them. It's that tough love concept again.

"That makes me think about something I learned about myself from this research," I say. "Several times, I've felt frustration that things aren't changing more rapidly than they are."

Alan responds, "I always get frustrated when things don't change rapidly. I think that's part of our personality."

"Yeah," I say. "I had that realization as I've been thinking about this research. I have a personality to fix things and fix them *now*. In a big way. I had a realization in one of the interviews that in a previous career I used to do life coaching to help clients set and reach goals. I have to admit I actually lost some clients because I pushed them too hard. They weren't ready to move as quickly as I wanted to encourage them to move. Rather than changing as rapidly as I was encouraging them to, they dropped the coaching. I admit, I have felt frustrated that things have not moved more quickly with this family, and I just wondered if you could talk about that. Is it on purpose that things haven't moved more quickly, is it by design, are you being strategic about how quickly you're moving things?"

"Strategic?" Nancy repeats.

It occurs to me that maybe I'm the only one who thinks things are moving slowly, and I'm trying not to sound like I'm criticizing them. "For example, Mrs. Stewart was going to move forward on the driver's license and nothing happened. Or movement on the house. A lot of other times, things have moved forward, and then they stop. Maybe this is normal with people in transition."

Nancy answers. "One thing is the way we measure change. When you're talking about the house moving forward, I look at it completely differently. Moving forward might be realizing, okay, if you really want a different house, then you're going to have to do some things to this house. You're going to have to get a checking account like we talked about and establish some credit, 'cause they pay in cash. They do pay, but they have no way to let people know that. Moving forward might be mentally moving forward, and it doesn't show on the outside. Also, moving forward, not compared to where other people are, but compared to where they were. I can tell you that progress might not seem like much, but we're talking about somebody who lost two sets of children. We're talking about somebody who lost their house and apparently was living in their car. Somebody that didn't have a caring relationship before that they were able to sustain. Where we might measure by our standards may be very different if you look at where they were. That's how I've adjusted my measurement. I really do think that some of what she wanted was a fairy godmother. That's not how it works. Nobody bought me a house. If you really want a house you might think about going to work. Your children are old enough to be unsupervised certain hours 'cause your husband's home. There's free checking accounts all over now, if you really want to do it. But if you don't really want to do that much, you might not really want it that much. You might just want somebody to figure out how to get it for you."

I'm amazed at how compelling her argument is for, basically, not helping.

Alan agrees. "She's so much better at that stuff than I am." He turns to Nancy. " 'Cause I think you're right on target with this family. That helping and not helping, or reframing what should be done, it's very possible that they may not do that. The reality is, though, that unless they do that, they ain't getting nothing, unless some benefactor gives it to them. I think you're very accurate in leading the team with the idea that you need to do these things differently. Basically, you need to jump through the hoops that our society has. Reminds me of the discussions I've had with my son over the last couple of years."

"Such as what?" I ask.

"Get a job," he says. "Get a checking account. Get a couple of credit cards. Run 'em up, but don't run 'em up too much, so you can pay them off, and make sure you pay them off. My son actually paid attention, and now he has this great credit rating. But it's very different from saying 'okay, let's work on getting you a new house.'"

"Very, very different," Nancy agrees.

"But don't they need to be told what steps to take?" I think.

"But it's what they need to do, if they're going to be self-sufficient in this society," Alan adds. "So let's go back to this house thing. There's other things to consider. We won't be around forever to help them, maybe not past this year. Don't forget the long-term medical issues. Mom and Dad are not old. They could be around for another two decades."

Nancy nods her head. "The other thing that has occurred to me is that she's all excited about moving to Plant City. She doesn't drive. There's no busses that go out there." Wow. This whole conversation is bursting my bubble. Now I wonder whose dream this is, anyway. I hate it when reality interferes with dreams.

"Which goes back to the driver's license. That represents empowerment for this family. Or self-sufficiency," Nancy says.

I just have to put in another plug for a house for the family. "You know, Mrs. Stewart has said that she could earn money doing her crafts. If she had a bigger house, she could make crafts and sell them."

Nancy argues with me. "Yeah, but this family has lived in housing projects. If you want to compare not having a house on your own and having a house on your own, to living in a housing project—that's what I'm saying. You've got to look at where they came from. She had the wherewithal to help her father-in-law figure out how to get that house. She had the wherewithal to help the church figure out how to put a new roof on it. She had the wherewithal to figure out how to get the paint. I'm saying that's compared to not having anything that you own—a place to live in, a car, enough food."

"She's also functioning better than she used to function," Alan adds.

"They pay their bills," Nancy adds.

"They have less than $4,000 left on their house," I add.

"When we first enrolled this family, a couple of people told us, 'don't work with the family at all, because they have chronic needs and you're not going to ever help them,'" Nancy remembers. "But I don't think that's true. Then they told me that I wasn't a good match for the family and that we really needed to hire somebody who could relate to the family on their terms."

Alan smiles. "Oh, that's right. We had that sophisticated Nancy conversation again." How very fascinating. I had no idea if I'd be able to bring that subject up with them.

"Actually, I've wondered about that," I say.

Alan responds. "It's not the family; it's the system people that you have to overcome this prejudice with. There are a lot of people that see Nancy as sophisticated."

I protest, "That's not a bad thing!" I think of my own self-image as a klutzy, nerdy, awkward person. I'd like to be thought of as sophisticated.

Alan continues, "High-class. Because of that they don't trust or believe that she has the ability to connect and have people be comfortable with her. That ain't true. It's not being culturally competent for the professionals."

How very interesting. "That's true. How does that factor in?" I ask, "'Cause I think that your culture does factor in to the way you relate to the families. This came out loud and clear in my interview with Mrs. Stewart the other day. She was talking about team members who don't understand her culture. All of a sudden I became very self-conscious about the car I drive and the clothes I'm wearing, and it occurs to me that to her, I'm the college girl. You know? I'm suddenly very aware of the way she sees me. I don't think it's purely in a positive way."

"Yeah, I've had confrontations with people in the system. Someday I'll wear a T-shirt and a pair of gross sneakers, and then they'll finally see it doesn't make a difference," Nancy offers. It occurs to me that she'd probably look sophisticated in a T-shirt.

I ask, "So what do you do? How do you deal with that?"

"It's probably a saving grace to me that I don't think about it very much," Nancy says, "because then I'm not self-conscious about it. Families have never had a problem with working with me."

"You just connect to them on the level of humanity?" I suggest.

"I do. We might be looking at something that we hope for or wish we had that's not the same, but the feelings of it are just the same." So she connects at the level of common feelings.

"How do you let the family know that?" I wonder. I'm thinking of how Mrs. Stewart claimed that the team can't understand her life and her stresses.

"I really am interested in what they're trying to say," she continues. "It's not something that I just have to pretend. I really am interested. Maybe from all the years of therapy. I know that most people's hopes, their dreams, what they're afraid of, there's a huge commonality. There's may be a difference in the way we live, but as far as what our feelings are about things, we're not that different. I think that it wouldn't be honest to pretend that I was somebody that I wasn't either, 'cause then I think that would come through eventually."

I think back to my interview with Mrs. Stewart. "When Mrs. Stewart was talking about whether the team understood her and her culture, she was talking about the school people, I think. She didn't seem to be concerned about you understanding her. That's interesting." In terms of dress and mannerisms, the other team members, especially Peggy, seem to be much more in rapport with the family than Nancy. Yet it's the others Mrs. Stewart seems to have problems with.

"I don't know. It's just something I don't think about very much. I forget about it until people make me aware of it," Nancy says.

Alan says, "This is the first family that this has come up with in a while, so I think it's getting better."

I respond, "It's so obvious with this family because it's an obvious difference in socioeconomics between you and them. It's huge."

They nod.

I think for a moment. "I was recently watching the videotape of the first focus group. When you guys were doing the collage, Jane put a picture of a boat on, and made the comment, 'this is the kind of boat we have.' You made a comment back, 'we have a boat similar to this, too.' I noticed the comments because, as you know, I'm taking sailing lessons, and I'm dreaming about buying a boat. It occurred to me at the time that it's interesting that we're talking about owning a boat, when this family barely made it to the meeting. They had to hold out grocery money to ride the bus. I wondered if they would see the disparities as an issue, but they never acknowledged hearing it."

Nancy responds, "I still think that if there's a basic respect and caring for people and they know it, they don't automatically expect your life to be like theirs."

Alan smiles. "If I come to somebody with problems, I wouldn't want the person I'm getting advice from to clearly have the same problems I do, right? You'd like to think they're a little more together."

"Right," Nancy says. "They don't really want to hear about my electric bill."

"When I used to do marriage counseling, the first thing people always wanted to know was, are you married or divorced?" Alan adds.

Nancy laughs. "Just say, I'm in the middle of a divorce. That's always a good one."

Alan laughs and adds. "Right. Right. It's a really nasty divorce."

I laugh.

Nancy pauses thoughtfully. "I'm thinking about the house issue again. There still might be resources out there. I'm still in hope mode."

Alan nods. "We're not going to give up," he says. I feel hopeful again.

"But the other obstacle, really and truly, is they can't clean out this house," Nancy says, "and she won't part with any of this stuff."

"That's why she wants a new place," I comment. "She sees a new place as her not having to get rid of stuff."

Alan says, "I was going to take a real estate person there and have them say, 'okay, you want a new place, you can't sell this one the way it is.'"

Nancy agrees. "They've got to sell that house. That's reality. They can't get into a better house without selling that one."

"I go back and forth with this thing," Alan says, "but I actually talked this weekend to a guy down the street from me who's a realtor, and they actually could sell that lot. They just wouldn't get a lot of money for it."

Nancy adds, "I was real upset after I talked to a mortgage broker, and I told the Stewarts, 'these are the reasons you don't have credit, because you use cash.'"

"We had this conversation, too," Alan interrupts.

"I said, 'I talked to a mortgage broker. You're not a first-time home buyer. You would have to sell this house to do that. You'd have to do certain things. You don't have a credit history because you pay everything in cash. If you really want to do it, you've got to think about this.' I was up front with her, and she took it really bad. I said, 'you know, another way you can have some income is get a job.'"

"You were very honest with her," Alan observes.

"Okay," I think to myself. "They are trying to take them through the steps."

Nancy continues, "I said, 'your children are old enough to let you get a job or do something with your skills of creativity, or combine both of those things to make some income.' If they're only willing to live on SSI, then that's the reality. But you have to get more money."

Alan sits forward and pauses for a minute. "You know, you've given me some ideas."

"What ideas?" Nancy asks.

"We still can go into this family team meeting with helping this family with getting a new house."

"But Alan," Nancy argues. "this is a long-term goal. Maybe five years out. We're going to have them in five years?"

"No, we won't," Alan responds, "but we can certainly help them to make up and start a plan. It's going to take them several years to get a new house. Realistically."

"By then the kids will be gone—they won't need a new house."

"Yeah, they will. The next bad storm that comes, this house is going to be gone. It's falling apart. Thank God we haven't had a hurricane." Alan turns to me. "They didn't have a house. They lived in public housing, and for a while they were homeless, so to own their own home and to be even talking about being able to sell a piece of property that's paid for, it's a pretty good place to be compared to where they were. Give them time, give them credit, give them some extra income, and they'll have the house paid off. Four grand is a lot of money when you're talking about this family and their house. Then they could actually achieve a goal. It's worth talking about, but we certainly have to get more realistic."

I feel more hopeful already.in all kinds of ways.

I think about Nancy and Alan's advice. What are their take-aways? Meet frequently as a team. Let the decisions be made at the team level, and make sure the family plays a strong part with a strong voice in those decisions. Let the team provide structure and direction. Keep frequent contact with the family so they always have hope of things getting better (short term and long term). Focus on changing the future. Relate to the family; show them you care. Talk, support, and *do*. Be honest and realistic. Be responsive—be *there*—be available to them. Separate judgment from diagnosis. See through their problems to find strengths. Practice cultural competence by balancing the fine line between respecting their culture and helping families work toward where they want to be in the future. Remember pain can bring about change. Be realistic about how you measure change. Connect at the level of humanity—common feelings, hopes, dreams, fears.

CHAPTER 8

Blended Voices: Constructing a Future with Hope

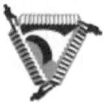

Transformed

It's been over a month since the team has met, and we greet one another like old friends. We're back in the time-out room at Washington, but it has been transformed since the last time I was here. The chaotic disarray of student and teacher desks has been replaced with matching tables and chairs, all lined up in neat rows. The room is spotless, and a colorful mural adorns one wall. Mrs. Stewart is resplendent in a calf-length, peach-colored, linen dress embellished with a hand-embroidered turquoise butterfly. Her hair is adorned with a beaded cap, and this is the first time I've seen her wearing make-up. Black fishnet hose peek out from above black ankle boots. Just as my friends and I say about ourselves when we get dressed up to go out, "she cleans up very nicely." She looks really good.

"You finished the butterfly!" I acknowledge excitedly, pointing to the embroidery on the front of her dress.

She nods proudly.

"It's beautiful! Look at how much work you've put into that!" I am truly impressed. The design is intricate, and there must be thousands of individual stitches involved. "I'm so glad you wore it!"

"I told you I would!" she says.

I've been working with this team for over a year, and it occurs to me that this final focus group is a graduation of sorts. I wonder what turning point this group meeting will be for her. Or me, for that matter.

I nod to Maggie to begin the videotape as we all settle down at the table. I pull my agenda out of my briefcase.

"I actually have an agenda today," I begin. "The first thing we're going to do is that collage, and then the sentence completion. We did them both in the first two focus groups, and it's been very interesting to see how they've changed. In the last focus group, you told me some questions that you wanted to ask, so I put those on the agenda. Then I'm going to go over my preliminary findings, and I want your feedback. Last I want to see what findings you think we should be coming up with, because I really see this research as a group effort. Are there any questions?"

Peggy nods. She's dressed, as always, in a tan polo shirt over black slacks. "Do we get to call you 'doctor' yet?"

I smile at the thought. "Not yet, but soon, I hope!" I open my mouth to continue but pause as the door opens and Warren enters. I had invited him to the meeting but hadn't really expected him to attend. For months he'd been too sick to be involved in the team. Despite his clearly having lost a large amount of weight, he looks great.

"Warren!" A chorus of voices echoes throughout the room as people jump up to shake his hand and bring him a chair. "It's so great to see you!"

Mrs. Stewart jumps up to give him a big hug.

"Welcome back!" I say warmly.

He smiles at me and makes himself at home at the table, looking as comfortable as if he'd never been absent.

I continue with the instructions. "Today's collage represents this team as it is today. In the last focus group, you said you wanted me to take part in creating it, so I'm going to."

We move to another table and get to work as we pull out construction paper, glue sticks, scissors, and magazines. The room falls into a hum of activity and friendly chatter as people cut, laugh, and share supplies. I'm astonished at how much fun I'm having joining them. The collage builds as we add a second sheet of poster board since our masterpiece has become too large for just one sheet. I'm amazed and excited at the change in the team since the first time we did this exercise.

Warren and Alan work on one end of the table, as Peggy, Jane, the Stewarts, Nancy, and I work at the other. The conversations ebbs and flows as people work and playfully fight over scissors and magazines.

Crossing Boundaries into the Future

A disarray of pictures, words, colors, and headlines forms as magazine scraps with cut edges, jagged edges, and torn edges are glued up, down, and diagonally.

Tiger Woods peers in the distance above a headline, "To Accomplish More, Sometimes You Have to See Less." Headlines proclaim, "Certain Restrictions Do Not Apply"; "Hunt. Gather. Action! One Goal: Victory!"; "One Intimidating Hauler!"; "Wanted: More Speed"; "Our Fleet Just Got a Whole Lot Faster"; "Secret Emotions: The Feelings You Don't Dare Share"; "Hocus Pocus"; "How Did We Get Here?"; "Some People See a Problem. Others, an Opportunity to Triumph"; "Taking the High Road"; "A Closer Look"; "Rock and Roll"; "Devotion to Duty"; "It's about Everything"; "Prepare Yourself"; "Go Off Road, but Stay On Track"; "Joie de Vivre"; "Journey"; and "Some Things Can Always Be Counted On."

A boat is partially covered by the headline "50 Years in the Water and No Signs of Wrinkles Yet." There's a guy on a motorcycle, and a guy on a skateboard. Guys swimming a race, and pictures of race cars. An old woman "Just Beginning" and a baby "Learning." A kid with a fish, and a kid underwater. Two young boys playing with fathers. Two pictures of people cooking, a woman making pottery, and a giant sequoia with huge roots.

I take a minute to look over the array. "What do we have here?"

The group takes a collective step back and looks. Mr. Stewart speaks first. "'Certain Restrictions Do Not Apply.' In friendships there are no restrictions."

Interesting, I think. "So, you're thinking that you've crossed boundaries to become friends?"

Mr. Stewart smiles. "Yes, we know one another now. We didn't know one another before."

Alan, dressed in his usual Hawaiian shirt and khakis, takes a swig of soda. He points to a picture in the center of the poster. "I have a picture of a young child and an older woman that represents this team, the old and the new. This guy is wondering what's going to happen in the future. This other picture is one of a parent and a child, very joyous, because I think that's the way the future is going to be."

Hope, perhaps, I wonder.

Jane points to an aerial photo of a winding road next to a headline, "Prepare Yourself." "We have to prepare ourselves; it's still a long and winding road. It's going to take character."

Peggy speaks next. "I have a lady doing pottery. The future is like a work of art. I want the Stewarts to remember the joy of living, which is not always easy."

Alan comments, "That was eloquent. I'm impressed." Everyone nods.

Mrs. Stewart points to the poster. "This says, 'Hunt. Gather. Action. One Goal: Victory.' All these together are what we are trying to do as a team. Even if we go off the road, we are still on the track that we started. No matter how hard it may be, we get to our ultimate goal, which is victory." She curtsies to an imaginary audience as the team nods in appreciation.

Nancy, looking professional in her linen jacket over lime sweater, points to a picture. "This represents the team—all the ingredients that get mixed together. Something new comes out of it; something better than all the separate ingredients. Everyone is different, and we all bring different things to the mixture. You put all this stuff together and something good comes out of it."

She points to another picture. " 'Some Things Can Always Be Counted On.' We have always come together to look at how things can be the best they can, how we can help the whole team and the family in doing all that we can. Something good is happening as we reach out to one another."

Several people smile approvingly.

Warren points to another picture. "This shows how determination will eventually pay off. The trees here are beautiful, and they stay that way."

Peggy answers next. "I put down 'Rock and Roll' because I do think we get a little rocky sometimes, but we roll right along. Another one I put down is 'It's about Everything,' because it is. Sometimes it might just be about Kevin and what he's doing that day, or it might be about what's happening in the home, or on campus, or in the mental health center, everything." She looks around the table at everyone listening intently. "This is my first experience with working with a team, so I thought, how did we get here? I see the team as its own identity at this point."

She points to "Wanted: More Speed." "This is my frustration. I would like to see things move a little faster sometimes."

Warren gestures toward the poster. "Everybody is here, and we all have different backgrounds, understandings, education, and cultures, but this lets us accomplish more. Sometimes we'll see Kevin as a young tiger being trained and developed to be an outstanding person. That takes the work and collaboration of all of us here. We're really focused on his development."

I take my turn to speak. "This is so much fun for me, because I've facilitated this exercise many times in focus groups, but I've never helped build the collage. I put up this one that says 'Take a Closer Look.' It's a kid swimming under water. This team represents a closer look at how to help Kevin and the family. I see a real focused, concentrated effort in what this team is doing.

"'Taking the High Road.' One of the things that struck me as I went through my research is the way every single member of this team is so strengths-based. In another research project, I've studied 118 team meetings over the last three years, and I have seen so many teams in which members are negative throughout the entire meeting. Yet every single one of you is taking the high road and remaining focused on strengths. That has impressed me."

I point to a headline, "Hocus Pocus." "I do think it takes a little bit of magic along with everything else to achieve what you want. 'Secret Emotions or Feelings You Don't Dare Share.' I think there has been a lot of sharing and self-disclosure, but also I think there are some things you guys still aren't saying to one another. I think there are some secrets among you. This child holding up his hand in victory. We have seen successes with Kevin, and there are things that he—and you—can be proud of that he's accomplished."

I point to another headline, "He May Not Remember His First Drive, but You Will." "It's a father and son driving. This team is really encouraging Kevin and his family and helping them to accomplish things that they will remember forever. There's one more, somebody water-skiing with a tow rope. I really like this as a metaphor of still holding on to Kevin. You haven't let him go, set him out there, and dropped him off on his own. You're still holding his hand, giving him a rope to hold to. I think that's a nice metaphor."

I'm pleased at how well the meanings described in the poster fit in with my analytical opinions, and I'm surprised at how I was able to find pictures and headlines that illustrate many of the points I wanted to make regarding what I think the team is constructing for themselves and the Stewarts.

We move back to our seats at the first table. As people bring food over from the deli tray I brought, I think about the take-away tips from the collage exercise. From the team's point of view, successful child and family teams will focus on the future and keep their eyes on the goal; focus on what they want—future strengths—rather than what they don't want; persevere but remember to have fun along the way; count on and reach out to every other team member. And, determination will eventually pay off.

Hope, Empowerment, and Support

"These are some sentences that I've asked you to complete in the last two focus groups, and I want to see how you answer them this time. To me, child and family teams are . . ."

Alan speaks first. "A way for folks to have assistance in meeting their own needs."

I read my next sentence. "What I like about being part of a child and family team is . . ."

Jane jumps in. "Collaboration."

"Listening," Peggy adds.

"We're having fun," Mr. Stewart says.

"I'm a member of this child and family team because . . ."

"I love Kevin," Mr. Stewart answers.

Alan and Warren nod.

"To this team, being strengths-based means . . ."

"Getting things done," Jane says.

"Working together," Warren adds.

Peggy says, "It helps them to set goals instead of getting bogged down in all the problems."

"To this team, empowerment means . . ."

Mrs. Stewart answers, "Working together."

Alan adds, "With the goal being that this family will be able to take care of themselves."

"Amen to that!" Mrs. Stewart says.

"To this team, having hope means . . ."

"Everything," Mrs. Stewart says. "The most important is having hope. That Kevin will go beyond his anger."

"To this team, family-centered means . . ."

Peggy responds, "The more we can assist with the family being okay, that translates to academic progress."

"If you are always centered on the family, the more empowering you will be," Mrs. Stewart adds.

"To this team, individualized care means . . ."

Mrs. Stewart answers first. "Doing what you need to do on your own but knowing that if you can't handle it, there are others waiting to take your hand and help guide you."

Warren and I nod at her response.

"Focusing on Kevin," Mr. Stewart adds.

"I agree," Alan says, with a mouth full of deli sandwich.

"To this team, being a team means . . ."

"Not being on your own," Peggy answers.

"Support," Alan adds.

"Hard work," Jane says.

"Yep!" Alan responds to Jane.

Nancy adds, "A lot of strengths."

"To this team, the future is . . ."

"I think it is now," Warren says, echoing his response in the first focus group. Heads nod.

"That is exactly what it is," Peggy says, "because whatever we do now is going to make a difference in the long run."

"If this team was a car, it would be . . ."

"A Ferrari, please!" Mrs. Stewart says with emphasis, still holding out for the luxury make.

The group laughs.

Mr. Stewart interjects, "That's right, because we've been together long enough to feel comfortable with one another and . . ."

Mrs. Stewart interrupts. "Something big enough to carry us all!"

"Yeah," Warren adds, "Something made by Mercedes." He gets up to get more food as Mrs. Stewart laughs with delight. Everyone is smiling.

Peggy answers. "I don't know why, but I'm thinking of a minivan. I think it's because our family's minivan lasted longer than any car than we've ever had, hauled more people around, had more stuff in it, and we lived in that car." All eyes are on her and heads are nodding in agreement.

I interject. "So you're saying that we keep going and going and going, and we're full of lots of stuff?"

"Yes," Peggy laughs. "It's an '88 but you can kick and kick it and it will still keep running."

"The major thing contributing to this team's success is . . ."

"Understanding," Mrs. Stewart says.

"Commitment," Peggy adds.

"Respect," Nancy says.

"Support," says Alan.

"The major thing I require from this team is . . ."

"Compassion," says Mrs. Stewart.

"Understanding," Mr. Stewart echoes.

"Collaboration," says Warren.

"Hard work," Alan adds.

Jane interjects, "You keep talking about hard work! There's that 'w' word again!" Everyone laughs.

"This team provides me with . . ."

Nancy says, "It would have to be support."

"Yes, I agree," says Alan.

"This team represents . . ."

"Kevin's best interests," Jane says, with a sincere look.

Mrs. Stewart agrees. "Exactly, what's good for him."

Alan adds, "I'll expand that—and the family's best interests." He makes intentional direct eye contact with Mrs. Stewart and she nods.

"My contribution to this team is . . ."

"Trying to explain Kevin," Mrs. Stewart says, pausing for a second before adding, "even though I don't do it very well."

"Patience and hard work, again," Alan says with a smile.

Mrs. Stewart interjects. "If you're going to get anywhere you've got to work. If you don't work, you might just as well hang it up."

"What this team does for me is . . ."

"Gives us an outlet where we can get our frustrations out," Mrs. Stewart answers, "but also get our ideas across of what might help."

Peggy adds, "This team honestly helps me worry less. When I work with families and children, I take that role seriously. Knowing that this team is involved with this family personally comforts me. I get a lot of reassurance that someone is working with this family in their best interest. I can't say that about a lot of agencies."

No Expectations

Jane takes a swig of water from her bottle as I move to the next agenda item. I'm impressed that we're still following the agenda rather than getting off track, as we did in the last two groups. "In the last focus group, I asked you, 'what questions would you like to ask?' Here's the first question you came up with, which I thought was a really good question: 'What were your expectations when you first joined this team?'" I look around, waiting momentarily for someone to answer.

"I didn't have any," Jane says, "because I'd never been in one. I had no clue."

"I thought it would be to help Kevin and his family see another way of living and to interject some resources into their lives," Warren says.

"Do you think that's happened?" I wonder.

"Oh, yes, it's happened," Warren says. "One of the questions I had when I came here today was how his behavior has been here at school as he made the transition."

"Oh, the progress is phenomenal," Peggy says.

Mrs. Stewart turns to Warren. "What you didn't see before you got here, Kevin had a minor outburst; it was a minor thing; a minor reaction."

Peggy sits forward. "I had an expectation of being able to get support from the parents in what the school was trying to do and support from the school for what the parents were wanting. My initial expectation was that the team would get the communication between home and school going a little better."

"Has that happened?" I wonder.

"Definitely!"

Alan speaks next. "My expectation was hard work!"

Everyone laughs at this fourth mention of the "w" word.

"I didn't know that, but it has been!" Peggy laughs.

Mr. Stewart says thoughtfully, "I thought it was going to be another sit down, discuss Kevin's problems, and then nothing happens, and we have the same problem."

Mrs. Stewart adds, "I had no idea what was going to happen. All I hoped for was the best. So far, Kevin seems to be doing better than he was. But there's still something we have to discuss—Kevin still thinks that he's going to go back to Memorial."

This is the first attempt to go off topic in this focus group. I'm amazed it has taken them so long. I decide to let them go in that direction for a few minutes.

Jane responds to her. "We have his IEP, his individualized education plan, it was due last week, I have a draft sitting right here. He's getting ready to apply for Level 5."

"As far as Kevin going back to Memorial, what do you think?" Peggy asks Mrs. Stewart.

Mrs. Stewart leans toward Peggy, making direct eye contact with her. "I don't think Kevin would do very well there. I think he's doing perfectly well right here. He's getting his grades brought up. He's learning a lot more about how to interact with others. If he was at Memorial . . ." she begins.

Peggy interrupts. "Then we need to think about how we're going to deal with that with him."

Mrs. Stewart responds. "He's going to get angry. But I don't think Memorial can handle him. Even with all his improvements, I still think he's out of their league."

Peggy says to Mrs. Stewart, "You do know that part of our evaluation is to help with that decision."

Mrs. Stewart nods in response. "I think Kevin is doing fine, right where he is. I would rather have him stay here for the last two school years."

"He's much higher functioning," Jane adds.

Warren leans forward. "I've got to jump in." His voice is loud to get attention from the other end of the table. "I think it's important for Kevin to have that as a goal. Going back to a mainstream school is his goal, going back to Memorial. If they can't handle him, they'll send him back, but if he can go there . . ."

Mrs. Stewart interrupts him. "I'm not going to tell Kevin you're not going to go back to Memorial. I wasn't going to tell him that. It would break his heart. I couldn't do that."

I note that they're trying to construct hope for Kevin.

Warren responds, "He's functioning, and he's trying to move to the next level."

Peggy speaks calmly and deliberately to get the attention back from Mrs. Stewart and Warren. "We'll be having a meeting at another time to discuss all this. Just so that you know, Washington High is evolving. The whole level system as Kevin knew it when he first came in is not necessarily the way the school is going to be run. We'll begin having some students graduate from here, and we're also getting a whole new facility with vocational education next year."

"Kevin would love that," Mrs. Stewart responds.

Peggy continues. "Either way, we'll sit down and deal with those issues in a team meeting. We don't want him to fail either way. We don't want him to blow up here and regress, and we don't want him to go to Memorial and fail and have to come back."

Voice on the Table

After a few more comments, I decide that it's time to get back to our agenda. "One of the questions that came up last time was, 'how do your communication styles affect the way you relate with the other team members?'"

Peggy moves toward the food table.

"In a positive way," Warren says. "I think the communication has been very good. Everybody has been able to express how they feel and not have to hold anything back. As far as helping Kevin and his family, you have to put it all out here on the table instead of under the table. When you put it on top of the table, everybody can see it and understand it. Then everybody can interpret it their own way and decide how they want to assist. Like you said, you know everybody in this group has been very positive, so it makes a difference if your communications are positive."

There is a long pause as people consider the question.

Nancy speaks next. "I think people are comfortable. Even things that are challenging or difficult, we can talk about them, and we know we're going to be listened to. There's not going to be a judgment in any way. It could even be seen as helpful."

"We're like a family," Mrs. Stewart says. I remember that several times she has mentioned how much she dislikes her family. I wonder what type of family she means, but I continue listening.

Peggy says, "I think that being in a team sometimes makes me think a little more before I speak. I think what I bring to communication is a task-oriented, direct approach."

"Is that good or bad?" I wonder.

"I don't know. You have to figure that out," Peggy answers with a smile.

"I would say that that's good," Alan says.

I continue, "I have a theory that I want to consider. I agree you're very open, but I also think there are some things you're not saying. I'd like you to write down what you have wanted to say to other people on this team but have not. I'm not going to read these comments out loud, but they may show up in my report."

Amid much nervous laughing and smiling, Peggy asks for clarification, "What are you doing with these?" I explain again.

Jane sits and looks at me for a long minute, while Alan finishes quickly. They write for several minutes, silently.

I fold the pieces of paper and put them inside my folder. Later, when I'm writing this chapter, I look at them. The answers are just as I had suspected:

"Don't be so critical and condemning about certain things."

"When does it stop when the situation is very one-sided? The people you are trying to help do not do their part. They want but don't give!"

"We still have let the family be dependent."

"I would like to tell Mrs. Stewart that she should avail herself of individual mental health services so that she can move on and be less traumatized by her past."

The emperor has no clothes, I think to myself. Even in a therapeutic context, social norms prevent us from saying some things that might be helpful to the team. I close my folder and look up around the table. "I'm not going to read these out loud, but I do want to ask you, what has stopped you from saying these things you wrote on the paper?"

"Respect," Mrs. Stewart answers quickly.

"Too personal to talk about in public," Peggy says.

"Timing," Alan says. "There's a time and a place for everything."

I move on. "Those are all the questions that came from you at the last focus group. Are there any other questions you want us to ask one another right now?"

Warren moves right back to problem-solving mode. "We were kind of getting to it earlier about this Memorial situation. Really, that is where his heart is at. To have trade schools and all this stuff here that Memorial doesn't offer is going to be a good opportunity. You just have to sit down and present it to him."

Peggy and Jane nod.

Warren continues. "Memorial has an ESE program also. There are some things there."

Peggy interjects. "I'd like to see you at the IEP—the individualized education plan—meeting."

Warren nods. "I'll come. I just need to know the date and the time. I'll be there."

"We need to decide, should we talk to him before?" Mrs. Stewart wonders.

Jane puts Mrs. Stewart's question aside and responds to Peggy. "I have his papers. We can discuss it right now, if you want."

Peggy suggests, "Why don't we set up another team meeting to come together for that?"

I interject, trying to regain control of the meeting to move back to my agenda. "Let's make sure before we leave today that you guys schedule a team meeting."

"Let's keep the IEP separate, and this can be our next team meeting's main issue," Peggy suggests.

Mrs. Stewart moves into decision-making mode. "Can I make a suggestion? How about the 4th of November, this coming week. We'd have the money to come back out here. We'd have to begin earlier than normal if that takes as long as I think it will, because we have to be back home before the younger kids get off their bus."

Peggy responds, checking her calendar, "The fourth at 11:00 would be fine."

I jump in, trying to help the team come to closure on the decision and attempting to regain control over the meeting. "Okay, so the fourth of November at 11:00 A.M."

The Moment of Truth

As they jot down that date, I open my notebook and move to talk about the research project. "As you know, I've been observing all of your team meetings and many of your interactions. In all, over the past ten months, I've attended five team meetings and four interactions between Alan and the Stewarts. I've conducted three focus groups and nine interviews with team members." I nod toward Alan and the Stewarts. "Even though I'm conducting this research, I value your knowledge also. I want to get your reactions to what I'm saying in my research is going on."

I pass out a handout as I continue. "There's something called dialectical tensions—opposite, contradictory tendencies—that everyone in relationships struggles with and negotiates through [Baxter & Montgomery, 1998; Bochner & Eisenberg, 1987; Cissna, Cox, & Bochner, 1989; Conville, 1998; Johnson & Long, 2002; Rawlins, 1983], and I think many of these are operating in this team."

Table 8.1 Dialogic Reconciliation of Dialectical Tensions

Struggles between...			Overcome the Struggles by...
Power	⇐⇒	Equality	Empathy
Difference	⇐⇒	Sameness	Engagement
Boundaries	⇐⇒	Relationships	Connection
Empowering (Enabling)	⇐⇒	Disempowering (Disabling)	Vulnerability
Control	⇐⇒	Emotionality	Possibility
Strengths	⇐⇒	Deficits	Support
Helping	⇐⇒	Not Helping	Blended Voices
Hearing	⇐⇒	Ignoring	
Hope	⇐⇒	Despair	Hope

I pause for a second. "I think the overriding struggle seems to be between hope and despair. As a matter of fact, I think that creating hope is essential to move you as a family and team forward. I think building hope is something you've worked for and have done in moments. It's hard to construct hope. When you were first working together, I saw a lot of despair and hopelessness. In today's meeting, I'm hearing sounds of hope."

I see several people smiling. "I think there are a lot of other struggles that are part of creating hope. I think you have to deal with issues of power and equality; feeling different from one another or seeing how you're similar; enabling and disabling—or disempowering and empowering; being emotional and maintaining control; focusing on strengths versus deficits; helping and not helping, and hearing and ignoring."

I glance up. Everyone is looking down at their papers. "A physician named Groopman [2004] describes hope as 'the elevating feeling we experience when we see . . . a path to a better future' [p. xiv]. Hope is about believing that a better future can happen and expecting that it will [Averill, Catlin, & Chon, 1990; Groopman, 2004; Snyder, 2000]. Having hope is also believing that you have the ability to influence outcomes in your life and that you have choices in life [Averill et al., 1990]. Hope is a spiritual idea, because it's about meaning, inner strength, and a determination to endure [Groopman, 2004]. Hope sets off a chain reaction that lets us move forward in the midst of adversity and in turns creates more feelings of hope" [Averill et al., 1990; Groopman, 2004].

I make eye contact with Alan, then look back down at my paper. "For many different reasons, hope results in positive outcomes for people with physical, mental, or social difficulties. Hope creates a placebo effect in which believing in a positive result can actually create one. Physically,

hope blocks pain receptors in the brain and changes neurochemistry
in the body, and hope is thought to contribute to the body's immune
response [Groopman, 2004; Richardson, 2002]. Greater hope is connected to better coping and recovery in patients, and, in fact, medical
patients who are hopeful have a shorter recovery time and a higher survival rate [Groopman, 2004; Snyder, 2000]. Hope can be thought of as
a protective factor that helps people deal with chronically stressful situations" [Groopman, 2004; King et al., 2003; Richardson, 2002].

I take a breath and continue. "Hope results in positive outcomes not
just for the hopeful person but also for those around him or her through
indirect communal benefits [Snyder, 2000]. Hope moves us away from
the problem-saturated past and present into a future with possibilities
[Groopman, 2004; Henderson, 2003] and both requires and enables us
to paint a picture of a positive future [Patterson, 2002]. Hope is a form of
discourse, or language, that generates possibilities for people in community. We create hope collectively by stating goals, developing steps toward
the goals, and by moving toward possibilities, by focusing on what can
be" [Barge, 2003].

I look up at the team. "At first, it seemed to me that all of you thought
the Stewart's situation was hopeless, and nobody seemed to know what to
do to move beyond that. When Alan joined the team, I think he helped
everyone see hope, and all of a sudden everyone started doing things that
moved the Stewarts, Kevin especially, in a positive direction."

I look at Alan. "Of course, as Alan reminded me, there's a fine line
between 'true' hope and false hope, and it's easy to construct false hope
if you're not careful."

I pause and look back down at my notes. "Hope has been described
as a feeling, a virtue, a personality trait, and a way of thinking and behaving" [Averill et al., 1990; Groopman, 2004; Snyder, 2000; Snyder &
McCullough, 2000]. "Hope is also created through communication"
[Barge, 2003]. I make eye contact with Nancy. "I think you created
hope by engaging in what communication scholars call 'dialogue'—
communication and understanding at a deep level of meaning [Cissna &
Anderson, 1998]. You did this through empathy, engagement, human
connection, vulnerability, creation of possibilities, social support, and
blended voices. So, for example, instead of focusing on whether Kevin
has strengths or deficits, you moved beyond that and focused on what
is possible for him. Dialogue inspires people to imagine possibilities and
take action toward them [Barge, 2003]. This study shows that strengths-
based language in many ways constructs hope in the system, and it also
shows how dialogue—beyond simply identifying strengths—builds hope
by reinforcing our interhuman connectedness, by normalizing the need

for help, and by reminding each of us that, in our humanness, we can and will survive."

I take a sip of water. "As you move through these struggles, you work through questions such as: Who gets to decide what's best for the family? Are the family and the rest of the team on the same side or separate sides? Who gets to talk and who gets heard? Are we looking ahead or back, toward positives or negatives? Are we looking at what is possible or what is impossible? Are we working together or separately? Is the family best helped by helping or not helping? I think that how you answer these questions determines if, and how, you give hope to the family and to the team."

I see several people nodding thoughtfully.

"As I said a few minutes ago, the next struggle I think you deal with is the issue of power and equality. Professionals typically hold more social power than the families they work with, and this power issue is something teams have to deal with. I think this team has done a really nice job with that."

I turn to Mrs. Stewart. "In a lot of ways, you have as much power as the rest of the team members, but I think the issue of sharing power is the tension that this team—and every team that works with families—continually deals with." I pause and wait to see if there is any visible reaction—whether Mrs. Stewart seems insulted or angry.

She's showing no reaction, so I continue. "I think the next struggle is between difference and sameness. The Stewarts are from a different culture than, I suspect, everyone else here." I shoot Alan a glance and a wink. "Well, maybe *almost* everyone else."

Again, I watch to see if there is any visible reaction or anger. Everyone is looking at me or down at their papers. They all seem to be listening intently. I continue to explain. "You've talked about how Kevin is different from his neighbors. I think there is this continual issue of being different and being the same. In some ways we are all the same and want the same things, but in other ways, we are very different."

I look around the table. "At the beginning of my research, it was as if there were three different subteams: the school team, the family team, and the Center for Children and Families team. You had limited cross-communication with one another. It seemed that boundaries between members prevented you from developing strong relationships with one another. However, you showed respect for one another and worked hard to give voice to one another in team meetings. Now, I think you've formed one team. As time has passed, relationships have begun to develop. You seem connected now. Mr. Stewart even illustrated that in the collage when he said that you've developed relationships."

No one has responded, not even with nonverbals, so I take a deep breath and continue.

"The next struggle is between enabling and disabling. This is a huge issue when you're receiving help. Are you being helped in a way that is empowering, or are you being helped in a way that is making you dependent on the system? I think this is a continual conflict. You talked about that in the last team meeting. Do you continue to give the Stewarts bus passes, which won't be available to help them in the long run, or do you help Mrs. Stewart learn to drive, which is a skill that will continue to empower her in the future?"

I move to the next item on my sheet. "Control and emotionality. There are control and boundary issues. I think that the boundary issues on this team are huge. I've seen role boundaries for many of us." I turn to Nancy. "In our interview, we talked about staying within the boundaries of being a therapist versus being a case manager. My boundaries as a researcher have come up throughout the research. I've tried to stay within those boundaries sometimes, and sometimes I haven't."

I gesture to Alan. "Alan had a role boundary when he was behind the camera and he broke through that boundary. Now look—he's sitting on this side of the camera, and stepping outside his assigned role helped to move things forward!" Alan smiles.

"In terms of control, the issue of setting boundaries for Kevin and controlling his behaviors is huge. You've come together to get on the same page to control Kevin and to control his emotions. You exhibit self-control, speak of restraining Kevin, create boundaries to control his behavior, establish rules to create safety, and try to calm him down. And I've seen many of us get emotional in team meetings. So there is a strain there between control and emotionality." I take another deep breath and wait to see if Mrs. Stewart seems upset at my mentioning emotionality in team meetings. Relief. She doesn't react.

"Strengths, deficits, and problems. This is a struggle for all teams and all people doing this type of work. I think you guys have been awesome at remembering that although Kevin has problems, he's also got strengths." I continue: "Focusing on strengths leads to hope. Hope draws on past experiences, borrowing strengths from your own past and from others who have endured their own trying circumstances [Groopman, 2004]. A scholar named Gergen says that changing the ways we talk about or interpret events will change behavior patterns. Continuing to see people in binaries—strengths or deficits, for example—will result only in superficial change. True change will result from finding new ways of talking about the world" [Gergen, 1999].

I pause. "I have to confess that through conducting this research, I've developed an appreciation for the difficulty of taking a strengths perspective. As I think back, I'm amazed and embarrassed at how many times I was critical of this team and your progress. I've often wondered why you haven't done more, or moved more quickly, to help the family. However, I've come to the conclusion that my tendency to make change quickly may not be in the best interest of a family. And I've also observed that letting a family move at its own pace and in its own direction may be more respectful than moving it at the pace I want it to go, in the direction I want it to go."

Several people nod thoughtfully.

"The next struggle is helping and not helping—when do you help, when don't you help? Determining what you help with, and what kinds of help to give, has been a tension," I say.

I'm past the findings that I thought would offend someone, so I relax slightly as I continue explaining. "Hearing and ignoring. I think people being heard is a huge issue. At times, many of you have struggled to be heard in the team meetings."

I still can't read their reactions. I move to my summary. "I think you deal with these struggles by a certain kind of behavior or communication called 'dialogue.' You show moments of empathy, engagement, and connection at an interhuman level [Buber, 1965]. You recognize that people are different, but we're all human beings, and we all want the same things and have similar values. You've been open and vulnerable to one another and accept and confirm one another as persons" [Anderson, Baxter, & Cissna, 2004; Cissna & Anderson, 1990].

I continue: "All of you are engaged in the problem-solving and planning process, and you're intentional about hearing one another. At times, you've shown a willingness to understand and even accept one another's opposition to your point of view [Hawes, 1994]. You've successfully overcome the struggle between strengths and deficits by constructing *possibilities*. You accept that Kevin has both strengths and deficits, that he is different in some ways and normal in others. Then you move beyond these differences and problems to work on what is possible, and when you do that, you create hope, for the family and for yourselves as a whole."

I see several people nodding and smiling. I move on. "Once you accepted your boundaries and worked around them, you began to create empathy. Rather than focusing on the tension between being the same or different, you were empathic toward the family. You don't gloss over the family's problems, but instead I've heard you say that 'they're doing the best they can.' You confirm the human goodness innate in the family and recognize your common human connection. You relate to the family at the level in which you're the same—the level of humanity. You also make yourselves vulnerable by self-disclosing personal information, emotions, and concern for one another. By being vulnerable to one another, you've been able to *both* express emotionality *and* maintain control.

"A wonderful example of interconnectedness and blended voice came about when you got on the same page and began treating Kevin consistently, with one voice. When you began interconnecting, you operated as a whole team but yet also maintained the individual voice of each team member. Rather than letting individual voices disappear into the dominant voice of the group, you created a multiple blended voice that hears all members' often conflicting voices, coordinating them but yet retaining their separateness.

"So, my point is that rather than focusing on the tensions, such as between being normal or different, or having strengths or deficits, you transcended those tensions through dialogue. Dialogue is not a continual process but instead shows up in moments, sometimes fleeting, sometimes messy, but always transcendent."

Finally, I'm done. The moment of truth. I turn to the team. "I want your feedback." I hold my breath.

Mrs. Stewart speaks first. "I think it's perfect."

I exhale.

She continues. "I think it describes everything that has been done and will continue to be done, until we get Kevin to the point where he no longer has such anger in him and will be more calm like he needs to be."

Alan speaks next and addresses the Stewarts. "The way you just said that, you talked in future tense. When we first met, you talked in the past. When you talk about hope, that is future stuff. You just gave a good demonstration about movement that is now focused on what is going to happen next, which I think is wonderful."

Peggy sits forward. "I'd like to talk a little bit about the differences and sameness. I see what you're saying, but at the same time I don't think there is a whole lot of difference. From my point of view, human beings are in large part a product of where they were born into, what they are used to, what they are in their family." She pauses and turns to Mrs. Stewart. "Where are you from originally?"

Mrs. Stewart responds, "I'm from here."

"What about your parents?"

"My father came from St. Louis," Mrs. Stewart responds, sitting forward toward Peggy and making direct eye contact with her, "and my mother was born here, full-blooded Indian, and my father's family was Irish. That's where I get my temper."

Peggy laughs. "Where did he come from in the country?"

"I don't know. My mom and dad, and his mother, are dead, so I don't have anybody that I can ask."

Peggy nods. "I'm going to share why I'm asking that. My family originally is from Tennessee, Virginia, and North Carolina, and I see in generations before me a lot of what I see in the Stewarts." I'm fascinated that Peggy, the person with whom Mrs. Stewart saw the most difference, sees similarity with Mrs. Stewart. I notice that Peggy and Mrs. Stewart are making strong eye contact.

"My father came from St. Louis," Mrs. Stewart responds, "and that's where his family came from. But where they were was very rural. We had chickens, we had a cow, pigs."

Peggy nods excitedly. "Exactly, that is what I'm seeing and when I see your lifestyle and the things that are important to you, I do see some of that like in my grandmother's generation."

"I'm a country girl, I do admit," Mrs. Stewart interrupts.

"There's nothing wrong with that," Peggy continues. "That's why I am saying, I don't know if we are all that different if we really sat down and traced where we're from and where we've been. I think humans in general living in certain circumstances would be very similar. Some people have no clue what people are going into and how they are living. As a social worker, I always try to put myself in their situation. If I had been born one of eight kids living in the projects, for example, what kind of decisions would I make? I just don't think we're all that different," she finishes.

This is my point, I think to myself. The team transcends differences by finding similarities! I'm so excited I almost interrupt, but I bite my tongue while Peggy continues talking.

A minute later, I continue with another thought that I direct to Peggy. "I also want to point out that when I had my interview with you, you were very strengths-based, and I was struck with your language, and with Jane's as well. It struck me how strengths-based and appreciative everybody on this team has been about everybody else, and how you guys think—as you just said, we do all have commonality."

"We really do," Peggy nods. "Because I know someone from rural areas, it reminds me of my roots. There's nothing wrong with that. I think that people who have been raised in the rural areas have a very strong sense of family, hard work, and making do with what you have."

Mrs. Stewart nods. "Making do," she echoes.

"I just think basically we're all human beings, and we all will act differently and be different depending on our environment. I try to get to the human being level as quickly as I can," Peggy adds.

"If I may interject an old adage, walk a mile in this person's shoes before you try to figure out who and what he is," Mrs. Stewart responds philosophically. She and Peggy are sitting forward toward each other, nodding and agreeing.

Warren interjects. "My relationship with everybody here is entirely the same. I don't see any separation. My focus was always to make sure that Kevin has the best possible services that he can get within the educational system. I always saw a connection with everyone else on the team, no matter who they were. I always saw that connection of how you could help to make Kevin and his family a better life."

I continue with my thoughts, "One of the other things that struck me is how very little changes have made huge consequences. For example, Alan joining the team had huge consequences. What Warren did in the classroom had huge consequences. I wonder if you guys can think of any other things that have had big consequences, big turning points in the team."

I'd call those times "turning points," and I can think of many: Peggy's comment to Mrs. Stewart in the first focus group; Mrs. Stewart's disclosure, in that same focus group, about her children who had been removed from her home; Warren's disclosure, also in that same focus group, about growing up in a foster home; the psychologist's report about Kevin; Mrs. Stewart bringing in examples of her crafts; and the new principal at Washington High. I wonder if they will mention these. Instead, they go in a different direction.

"If we go back to the very beginning of just having a team," Nancy says, "the very fact that we have a team had large consequences. Kevin doesn't see us as just a separate group of people that he knows. He knows that we all get together, and we've gotten to be a team, and we're all supportive of one another. That sets a very different tone than would just a bunch of separate individuals who all know Kevin and want to help him."

Alan responds next. "I would say that I think some level of sacrifice and also dedication made a big difference." He turns to the Stewarts. "The two of you spent a lot of time and effort getting to this very room here." Next he turns to Jane and Peggy. "Even though sometimes it probably seemed as though there were a million people calling you, the two of you stayed in here, and I think that took determination. Those things are very little when you take them separately, but when you put them together, this is major consistency, and it's huge." Now he turns to me. "I also think that your research had a lot of effect as the glue that's keeping this team together."

I take the bait, "Well, I was going to ask you about that. How has my research affected this team?"

"A lot," Nancy says.

Peggy adds, "It seems to me that we had to evaluate ourselves more. In a way, because we had to answer your questions, it was almost like a challenge to the team. We had to ask ourselves whether we *are* a team or not. Even though they were very nonthreatening questions, they were still questions that made you think. Thinking about it made us be more of a team. I'm a little worried about it ending, and I'm making sure that we all stay together and keep meeting. Because you really drove our schedule a lot."

Several heads nod. Peggy continues. "Keeping up regular meetings. Sometimes we'll schedule a meeting and then can't get together. Your research gave us more structure. And, it was an informal get-together, and we could always count on having," she turns to the Stewarts, "you two especially, at the table, every single time." She turns to me. "The scheduling and the structure."

Mrs. Stewart picks up the conversation. "It's like you put a mirror in front of each one's face and made us see ourselves as others see us, not the idea of our self that we have, but as others see us. You put that mirror image in front of our face and said, this is how others see you, not how you see yourself, how you really are."

I'm pleased that she thought the reflection was helpful to her and to the team.

Jane jumps in. "We have to look at ourselves as a team, as individuals and as a team."

Peggy addresses the Stewarts. "I think that the focus that also has been placed on your achieving and setting goals has made a difference. I see a different Mrs. Stewart at the table today than I did a year ago." She turns toward Mr. Stewart. "I think you're more articulate. You know what you're doing more. You're more self-confident. I think you've always been wonderful because you just are solid. You are always there," she turns to Mrs. Stewart, "so you have wonderful support. But I do see you as very much more relaxed. You know that old saying, 'if mama ain't happy, nobody's happy?' Mama's happy now. What the Center for Children and Families and this team have done with helping you, it is showing."

Mrs. Stewart nods. "Well, she's right about that. This is the first time I've ever showed off anything that I have ever made."

Wow! I never would have said that Mrs. Stewart had low self-esteem. What a statement!

"I couldn't even see to thread the needle," Jane affirms.

"It's the first time," Mrs. Stewart repeats.

"Well, I'm honored," Alan says to her.

"It's wonderful," she responds, in a surprisingly quiet voice. "All of you have made me realize that I do have stuff I can be proud of, not just producing children."

I notice that the table is full of affirming smiles and nods.

I continue. "Let's talk more about my interaction with your team. What was it like to have me involved?"

Peggy sits forward. "The videotaping bothers me, that's all. You've been wonderful. You've been flexible, staying together with us and everything. To get all of us in a meeting or get to any of us individually."

I respond with my own appreciation. "What you guys have done to accommodate your schedules for me, everybody is here at this meeting, and I am just so appreciative and excited." I pause. "So, how did my participation make you feel?"

"I really don't know," Warren says. "I'm glad you were involved. It created some structure on the agenda, and I guess it kept us focused on what we were trying to do. It's easy to get with teams and lose your focus and your direction, and then people start falling off by the wayside. When that happens, the parents get upset because they see no direction. Then, they see no hope, no end, no light, and they drop out. And the kid gets worse, because the parents have a negative attitude and the kid feeds into that and brings it back to school. I think that's probably one of the things that helped Kevin. Mom and Dad go home with a positive attitude, with reassurance, with some hope. They go home being able to see that there is a direction, that there are some resources out there. Kevin has to pick up on that."

Mrs. Stewart responds. "Well, I will tell you all something that I did, and I think it's a good thing. I figured out a way to give Kevin and Gary some privacy. I bought some clothesline rope and a tarp. I stretched it across the room and I took the tarp over it and now Kevin has his half, Gary has his half and they both have privacy. It seems to work very well."

There are lots of smiles and nods around the table. Empowerment in action, I think.

"What an excellent idea!" Alan says.

I continue, "Alan and Nancy, how have you felt about my involvement with the team?"

Nancy answers first. "I think for me it's been very positive. Backing up a little bit, your communication training, you taught us what teams were about and communication skills. We were always aware of the importance of the team with the family, but somehow the other dimension of you being here and what you're doing made us even more aware of really being a team. It created an awareness of our group as a team, a team effort."

I look at Alan. He says, "I feel fine."

"Okay," I say, and wait.

He turns to the rest of the team. "Cris and her data collectors have observed teams on this program for the last three years, so this is more normal than not."

I ask, "Would you say I'm a team member or am I an outsider?"

"I think you're a little of both," Mrs. Stewart says.

"You're an outsider looking in," Mr. Stewart adds.

Peggy says, "Initially, I had a concern because you were an outsider and because of the parents' right to confidentiality. I wanted to make sure that they were protected and you were not really a part of the team. My other personal reaction was, 'oh no, I just got one more person I have to talk to, deal with, schedule around.' I think that it has really been very helpful for me to have you here, because I do see more of a team kind of thing. I don't know if I were just on a regular team without you, if I would see it the same way. I think it has been really good training for me."

Alan adds, "I think that one of the things that's happened is that I've seen us keep more on track and more structured. I personally believe that you've always been a member of the team, because you influence the team, so you can't not be a member."

Last Words

I continue, "Okay, my last formal question. If you were writing up this research about what the team has been constructing and communicating for the past year, what would you say? What would your conclusions be? How did your team interact? How does your team communicate? How do you treat one another? What does all of this mean about the future of teams? What can we tell people?"

Jane sits forward. "It can work, it's not all just accusatory stuff, like you did wrong, and shame on you, and this is what you need to do, and you, you, you. It's more about all."

Peggy adds, "Because I'm not a teacher and I'm not an educator, I tend to see things differently. I think in the education system, we professionals tend to think we have it all figured out, and if the parents would just do such and such, everything would work. I think that the parent, on the other hand, sometimes comes to the table with the idea that the child is there eight hours a day, do what you got to do and fix him."

I see lots of nods. She continues. "So I think that the team approach really helps wade through all of that. In particular, I think what this team did with Mr. Camelini last year and his classroom situation was invaluable. I think that it helped him feel supported. I think it does make us kind of sit back and go, there is more than one way of doing something. I think that the parents also learn from the team. I just love it. I wish we could do this with every single one of our kids, but with the amount of time it just takes, we are out of time to do this."

I nod. "Yeah, I know that this approach seems to be awfully time consuming. And, it can be expensive in the short term, too, versus traditional treatment approaches [Bickman et al., 2003]. But if the alternative is to wait until the problem gets so serious that Kevin ends up in jail or a residential treatment facility, I think the cost to society is well worth it." I look down at my notes. "Research has found that placement in systems of care—teams like this— improved outcomes for children in the foster care system [Clark et al., 1996); improved delinquency behaviors of boys and increased the likelihood of permanent placement for older youth in the foster care system [Clark et al., 1998]; improved home behavior and the parent-child relationships among severely maladjusted boys ages 5–28 [Clarke et al., 1992]; and prevented placements in more restrictive educational and residential settings" [Eber, Osuch, & Redditt, 1996; Skiba & Nichols, 2000; Yoe et al., 1996]. I look back up. "So, even though the cost of treatment is higher, in the long run, the systems-of-care approach like this team prevents long-term societal costs such as the cost of foster care, hospitalization or incarceration, criminal activity, or welfare-related costs."

I see several people nodding. I continue, "You know, this research has strong implications for how professionals deal with families in crisis. Systems-of-care teams as a concept has a lot of potential for drastically changing the relationship between families in need and care providers. What seems to be missing from the description and definition of systems of care is a transcendent dimension that goes beyond superficial changes and creates 'second order change' in the system as a whole."

Alan smiles. "Then, Cris, what do you suggest a system of care should be like?"

"There's some recent research that suggests a version of systems of care called a Soft Systems Methodological Approach, or SSM. This version suggests that providers establish and maintain a focus on shared values and beliefs, shared responsibilities and actions, and flexibility in response to developing conditions [Hodges, Ferreira, & Israel, 2012]. There's also lots of research that supports the importance of culturally competent care. Other researchers focus on the importance of family-based and individualized care and agency collaboration, as this team has done [Miller et al., 2012]. I agree with them, and I think we've seen a lot of that in this team. I also think a system of care should foster dialogic relationships— deep interpersonal relationships in which families and informal supports have as powerful a voice as do professionals and service providers. I have a vision of service providers taking a coaching orientation to their care relationship. Rather than either doing or not doing things for families, they'll stand next to them, hold their hand, and teach them—one step at a time—how to set goals and take baby steps toward reaching them."

I pause and think for a minute. "Also, providers will let themselves be vulnerable—to developing a relationship at the interhuman level with one another and with the families they're helping. They'll appropriately share parts of themselves to develop rapport and model success strategies for families. They'll be open to possibilities—to radical changes in the families and in themselves and will be willing to suspend assumptions and judgments and see one another in new ways. Teams will understand society's role in the family's situation and, rather than judging family members for their problems, will help them find new ways of dealing with their issues by helping them dream of better possibilities for them. They'll also look inside themselves to understand how they are affected by the family's situation and how their own frames of reference influence their relationships with the families with which they work."

I look around the table and think of the many ways today's meeting was dialogic. "In a dialogic relationship, system-of-care partners will accept one another and recognize that we all have positives and negatives, needs and resources, strengths and deficits, and they will also help families recognize that. They'll create hope both for the families and for themselves by focusing on a positive future rather than past or present problems, on what can be done rather than what can't be done, on people's abilities to make a positive contribution to their world, and on the human spirit's ability to transcend problems." I pause and tap the table for emphasis as I read from my notes. "Hope, like dialogue, is transcendent. I think that moments of dialogue lead to moments of hope, and moments of hope move families forward into a future with enhanced health and well-being."

Peggy nods and turns to the Stewarts. "The fact that Kevin knows that you were very much supporting what is happening here at Washington makes all the difference. He knows that this is a group, it's not Mom and Dad against the teacher or the teacher against Mom and Dad."

As if on cue, Kevin's face appears in the window of the door. Mrs. Stewart comments first. "Kevin's outside," she says calmly. Warren stands up and goes to the doorway. He disappears out the door for a brief moment. We continue the discussion, and he rejoins us, with no more comments made about Kevin's appearance.

"What last words do you want to say in my research?" I ask the group.

Nancy answers, "It doesn't feel like a last word, because our team will continue."

Warren speaks. "I think it's been very positive the way we worked with Kevin's class and with his family life. Give them credit. Kids who do well, their parents are always involved in the education process. The other kids whose parents are not involved, who don't come to meetings, those kids suffer. They're dysfunctional, and they really run behind. Kevin's got support from the school, parents, the Center for Children and Families. Everyone's giving him boundaries. I can see a big difference." He grins. "He's walking differently. I'm really proud of him."

Jane nods. "When I look at his behaviors, he's doing extremely well. He still needs a little persuading from time to time, but he handles it much better than he did. All 15- or 16-year-olds have tizzies. He's handling it much, much better. He's come eons."

Everyone nods.

Jane continues. "I look only at what is. You can help only the future. You can't change the past. Go from there and do the best you can."

"What next?" Peggy wants to know.

"Well," I respond. "This focus group will be my closing chapter. I wanted you guys to have the last word."

I turn to Warren. "Your illness was an ethical challenge for me. I felt that I had permission to write about your interactions with the team, but I didn't feel that I had the right to write about your health problems."

"That's all right," Warren says, but I continue.

"Yet several people who read drafts of my manuscript wanted to know, 'what happened to Warren?' I didn't know what to say. Could I say that you were ill?" I ask.

"Say I almost kicked the bucket twice," Warren responds, with emotion. He turns to the rest of the table. "I'd like to explain where I've been. I've had kidney disease for the last 9, 10 years. The doctor was watching it, and everything was fine. I got an extensive physical several months ago, and my blood pressure was high. Then I started getting short of breath, and they found a spot on my heart. They took another blood test and found that I have an autoimmune disease, similar to lupus." I notice that everyone is sitting forward, listening intently. You could hear a pin drop.

He continues. "My blood pressure went up, and my kidneys shut down. I was rushed to the emergency room. I had fluid building up on my heart and then my lungs. I had two surgeries. I was in the hospital for 27 days. I lost 50 pounds. It was quite an experience. I was in the hospital wondering if I was ever going to leave. God's been real good. My family got closer together." He begins sobbing and pulls out a handkerchief from his pocket and wipes his eyes.

"How do you feel now?" I ask quietly.

"I feel wonderful!" he answers. "I've got dialysis three times a week." He wipes his eyes again. "It's amazing. There's a lot of people, they go in, they can't walk, they're hurting, paramedics bring them in and take them out. I go in on my own. I'm thankful."

"You've got to take care of yourself," Peggy admonishes.

Warren seems to struggle for words. His next sentence comes out in a rush of emotion. "I'm going to *die!*" he says, with a strong emphasis on the word "die." "I might as well do what I want to do." The room is speechless. "I can't sit home and wait. For the last year I haven't been doing much of anything. Now I'm going home to California for two weeks—I can get dialysis out there. I'm going to Taiwan, I can get dialysis out there. I'm going to start traveling again. I can't stay still. Guess I'll die in an airplane. I'll die doing what I want to do rather than just sitting back and waiting to die. I feel good. My dialysis is not that difficult; I get a lot of paperwork done during the 3½ hours."

The team is exchanging admiring glances. For his—courage? Hope? "It's been a blessing," Warren continues. "I'm glad to be back working." He wipes his eyes.

The Stewarts have to catch a bus, so the meeting breaks up. Warren gives me a huge bear hug. I'm surprised at the level of emotion I'm feeling. I feel a mixture of gratitude, excitement, compassion, and pride for the group and me, for how far we've all come.

My reverie is interrupted when Jane whispers to me, "Here's a last word—when are we going to Disney World?"

I laugh.

Disney World—the land of dreams and possibilities. Maybe, in a sense, we've already gone.

As I walk to my car in the warm sun, I feel the heat on my face as I lean back and exhale deeply. I close my eyes and think of my favorite Bible verse, from Jeremiah: "For surely I know the plans I have for you, says the Lord, plans for your welfare and not for harm, to give you a future with hope." Regardless of how black the clouds look some days, through relationships and community, we can come together to construct hope.

CHAPTER 9

Children's Mental Health
Practice Considerations

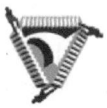

Systems of Care in Children's Mental Health

The children's mental health care system studied in this research is a community-based program providing mental health services to children with Severe Emotional Disturbances (SED). This project is one of over 125 programs around the country funded since 1993 by a grant from the Child, Adolescent, and Family Branch of the Center for Mental Health Services (CMHS) in the Federal Substance Abuse and Mental Health Services Administration (SAMHSA), with the goal to develop and encourage system-of-care practices in children's mental health (Lezak & MacBeth, 2002; Stroul, Blau, & Sondheimer, 2008).

System-of-Care Principles

Children with SED typically have multiple needs and thus are served by multiple agencies and organizations, such as education, social service, juvenile justice, health, mental health, vocational, recreational, and substance abuse providers. The system-of-care philosophy is one in which all the children's mental health care providers in a community come together to provide services to children with SED and their families in a coordinated manner. The system-of-care approach also includes family involvement in which families of children with SED are treated as full participants in the planning and delivery of services. Cultural and linguistic competence, the consideration of the unique needs of people from different cultural back-grounds, is also a critical component of the system-of-care philosophy—as are a wide variety of services across multiple domains: least restrictive service provision; interagency coordination; early intervention, and some-times individualized services in the form of flexible funding support (Rotto, McIntyre, & Serkin, 2008; Stroul, Blau, & Sondheimer, 2008; Stroul & Friedman, 1994).

This approach is a philosophical approach based on systems theory. Individual children are viewed systemically, within the context of their physical, mental, and emotional systems. They are also viewed within their family system, as well as within their community system, including extended family, neighbors, clergy, and other informal supports. In addi-tion, their care services are viewed systemically, within the holistic array of multiagency, multidisciplinary services (Hodges, Friedman, & Hernandez, 2008; Stroul, Blau, & Sondheimer, 2008; Stroul & Friedman, 1994).

The system-of-care philosophy is built around three core values: (1) a focus on the needs of the child and the family; (2) care provided in the child's and family's local community, in the least restrictive environment; (3) cultural and linguistic competence, which means that the child's and family's language, culture, and ethnicity are taken into account by provid-ers (Stroul, Blau, & Sondheimer, 2008; Stroul & Friedman, 1994). The 10 principles, or basic beliefs, of a system of care are these (Stroul, Blau, & Sondheimer, 2008, p. 6):

1. Children with emotional disturbances should have access to a com-prehensive array of services that address the child's physical, emo-tional, social, and educational needs.
2. Children with emotional disturbances should receive individualized services in accordance with the unique needs and potentials of each child and guided by an individualized service plan.
3. Children with emotional disturbances should receive services within the least restrictive, most normative environment that is clinically appropriate.
4. The families and surrogate families of children with emotional distur-bances should be full participants in all aspects of the planning and delivery of services.
5. Children with emotional disturbances should receive services that are integrated, with linkages between child-serving agencies and

programs and mechanisms for planning, developing, and coordinating services.

6. Children with emotional disturbances should be provided with case management or similar mechanisms to ensure that multiple services are delivered in a coordinated and therapeutic manner and that they can move through the system of services in accordance with their changing needs.

7. Early identification and intervention for children with emotional disturbances should be promoted by the system of care in order to enhance the likelihood of positive outcomes.

8. Children with emotional disturbances should be ensured smooth transitions to the adult service system as they reach maturity.

9. The rights of children with emotional disturbances should be protected, and effective advocacy efforts for children and youth with emotional disturbances should be promoted.

10. Children with emotional disturbances should receive services without regard to race, religion, national origin, sex, physical disability, or other characteristics, and services should be sensitive and responsive to cultural differences and special needs.

Ramifications of Research

This longitudinal, qualitative, case study research yields many findings that have actionable ramifications for mental health care providers involved in children's mental health teams and systems of care, as well as for providers in other helping professions.

Specifically, this chapter looks at five key areas of practice considerations that make a positive difference in implementing systems-of-care principles, empowering clients, and improving outcomes for children and families: (1) using strengths when working with clients; (2) using communication that is empowering and enabling for clients; (3) developing an appropriate therapeutic relationship with clients; (4) using meeting facilitation skills to set boundaries and balance flexibility and structure on the team; and (5) facilitating meetings and interactions so that the family's voice is heard and acknowledged.

1. Strengths Orientation

One thing that's clear from this research is that a strengths orientation to clients goes far beyond a rote listing of "what is mommy good at?" although that may be a good place to start. A strengths orientation that makes a difference for clients and providers is a philosophy that focuses on people's personal and environmental resources, rather than on their problems or deficits, and that focuses on positive possibilities, rather than on fears and challenges. A strengths philosophy is a belief that, regardless of first impressions, everyone has positive things in their past, present, and future that can transcend their problems and improve their functioning. I'd define a strength in this context as "something positive within the child, parent, family, team, or environment that can be used to move [the person] forward toward greater health and well-being" (see Davis et al., 2012).

This area is a challenge in the human service field. It's not that providers wish the worst for the families they're working with, but it is frequently very difficult for them to see family and child strengths in the midst of the deficits, problems, and challenges that are bombarding the team. Child and family teams (and other therapeutic relationships) don't come together because the family is doing well. They come together because of the family's problems, and if that fact remains the main focus of the team, they will be unable to develop a strengths orientation. When we compare what one family has with what others have, or with what they don't have, deficits stand out.

Teams operating under system-of-care principles know they are supposed to identify strengths, but many simply do a rote listing of strengths before moving on to the "real reason" they are meeting—the child's problems. This activity may fulfill the "letter of the law" but definitely not the intent of the exercise. Teams make a positive difference for children, families, and themselves by using strengths as interventions or change agents. Family strengths are those things in the family's values, culture, competencies, and interaction patterns that help them to function, even in the midst of problems (Dunst, Trivette, & Mott, 1994). A strengths-based approach carries with it the assumption that all people are either currently functioning well or have the capacity to learn how to function well (Dunst, Trivette, & Deal, 1994). Thus, this approach has the goal to develop a family's strengths rather than fix their problems and to help people to help themselves as they build on what they already have (Dunst, Trivette, & Deal, 1994; Dunst, Trivette, & Mott, 1994; Durant & Kowalski, 1993).

In systems of care, child and family treatment teams conduct what is called a "strengths assessment"; the purpose of this assessment is to help teams to find out what resources are available and what potential interventions can be used in a strengths-based plan. Often this assessment is simply a recitation of strengths, but teams are most effective when they specifically tailor a strength to a family's specific plan or needs. Tying strengths to needs also ensures that the family and the team agree on what the actual needs are—a lack of consensus on needs is a source of family-team conflict (Dunst, Trivette, & Deal, 1994).

In this and other research (see Davis et al., 2012), colleagues and I have identified 11 key ways that strength-based communication can be used in work with children with SED, their families, and their mental health care providers. This typology of strength-based communication is helpful to remind service providers of many strengths that they typically overlook. Thus teams can talk about child and family positive traits; child and family positive behaviors; child and family interests; child and family resilience; child and family dreams or possibilities; available family and team resources; borrowed strengths; past or historical strengths; environmental strengths; positive feelings, attitudes, and values; and hidden strengths.

When a provider communicates about traits, he/she talks about skills or things in which the child or family (or team members) excel, such as Kevin's math ability or Mrs. Stewart's sewing skills. Mrs. Stewart is competent at seeking help for her family and in communicating in a way such that her family's needs are heard.

Providers communicating about positive behaviors remind the team about specific behavioral examples of strengths, such as when Mr. Stewart purchased and installed a new bathtub, when Mrs. Stewart embroidered the dress, and when Kevin buckled down and did well on his assignment.

Communicating about interests entails talking about things a child or family is interested in doing that would move them in a positive direction, such as Mrs. Stewart's interest in crafts. (Interest strengths are often manifested in behavioral strengths—when a person is interested in something and then does it.)

Sometimes teams remind themselves about their (or the family's) resiliency—a personality trait that enables a child or a family to have survived so far in the face of difficult life circumstances (Dunst et al., 1994; Richardson, 2002). Examples of resiliency include the persistence of Mrs. Stewart in obtaining help for her family and Jane's ability to remain calm in the midst of ongoing crisis.

Teams can look at dreams, or what I call "possibility strengths." This type of communication looks ahead to the solutions, goals, or dreams set in the future toward which the family and the team are working. These types of strengths use imagery to show the family what they have to look forward to or toward what they can work (Berg & DeShazer, 1993; Fanger, 1993). Possibility strengths move the family out of a present-time focus, which is often laden with problems and deficits, into a future-time focus, which may be seen as a time of hope. Possibility strengths are stated in the positive and answer the question "what will it look like when things are better?" They move the team's communication and attention away from problems or deficits and negative, destructive behaviors toward thinking about positive, concrete alternatives. In practice, they move the team out of an either/or orientation that limits their options to a both/and orientation that opens up options and solutions (Lipchik, 1993). The more specific and tangible a possibility strength, the better able the team is to create a visual image of it. You can ask your family or client the following questions: What specifically do you want? What will it look like when you get it? Where and with whom do you want it? What will you be doing, saying, and thinking when you have it? Possibility strengths turn negatives into positives. A new home for the Stewarts would be a possibility strength.

Teams exist to provide resources for the family, and reminding themselves of these resources is another way they can communicate a positive direction for the team. Resources can be money, time, or knowledge available to help the family and team to achieve their goals. Mr. and Mrs. Stewart's, Alan's, and Warren's different kinds of knowledge of the system are resources. The assistance budget is a resource provided by the community mental health care system, and psychological testing is a resource that the school provides. Other types of resources include food/clothing and transportation, and environmental, medical, vocational, educational, recreational, emotional, cultural, and social resources (Dunst, Trivette, & Deal, 1994).

Strengths can be borrowed or taken from another person or from the intervention or treatment itself (Groopman, 2004). Warren's intervention with Kevin's classroom was borrowed from the other work he had done in other schools, and the school staff's success in controlling Kevin's behavior was borrowed from their experience with other children at their school.

Strengths can also be borrowed from the family's past. The Stewarts have a history of overcoming disability, homelessness, and family crises. They've done it before so they can do it again.

Strengths can be taken from the environment, like the fact that the Stewarts have a home with a mother *and* a father at home.

Strengths can also be a feeling, attitude, or value-attitudes or beliefs that are helpful for a family (or team member) to have. The Stewarts' desire to keep their family intact is a value strength.

Strengths can be identified that are hidden—things that, on the surface, look like deficits but could be turned into strengths. Kevin's aggressiveness could perhaps be a positive thing if he learned to channel it in a good direction.

Effectively communicated strengths give a family or a team hope, because they show that the family is good at something that can be used to help them; they orient the team toward a hopeful future; they remind everyone they're not in this alone; they provide resources, ideas, and suggestions that the family and team can use; and they remind everyone that they can accomplish their goals (Davis et al., 2012). Focusing on strengths reminds everyone that they are greater than their problems, and it gives a foundation on which to build goals and plans.

2. Enabling Communication

According to previous research (Davis, 2006, 2008; Davis, Dollard, & Vergon, 2009), communicating to caregivers and families in ways that empower rather than disempower them can be a challenge for mental health care providers. In the short run, teaching caregivers how to do something for themselves takes more time than simply doing it for them. As long as providers are burdened with high caseloads and impossible expectations, and as long as families remain in crisis mode when receiving help, it is very tempting to take those short-term shortcuts. This research shows that empowering and enabling communication is both possible and desirable. In the long run, teaching caregivers and families how to help themselves—how to find and process information; think in ways that move them away from deficit beliefs; navigate systems; perform essential skills and behaviors; and communicate with providers and systems in ways that get them what they need—gives them independence and hope for the future.

Steven Covey's "Time Management Matrix" (2004, p. 151) is a useful visual tool here. Table 9.1 shows his theory adapted for work with children and families. Covey's High Importance, High Urgency Quadrant (what I call the Reactive Quadrant) represents the things you need to do to help a family in crisis mode. If they're homeless, you need to find them a place to live. If the child is about to be kicked out of school, you need to react immediately and appropriately. However, problems occur when the family never moves out of this quadrant. Staying in crisis mode encourages more crises and eventually results in disempowering and disabling behaviors. As soon as possible, move the families into what I call the Proactive Quadrant, the quadrant in which goals are important but not urgent, such as getting more education or getting job skills training. Spending time in the Proactive Quadrant prevents time being spent in the Reactive (crisis mode) Quadrant. The other two quadrants are the Time Waster and Out of Control Quadrants, and Covey suggests that resources can be moved from these two quadrants to the Proactive Quadrant to enhance a person's chances of success (Covey, 2004, pp. 151–54).

In this research we see many empowering and enabling behaviors. We see many examples of team members acknowledging each of the Stewarts

Table 9.1 Important/Urgent Quadrant Analysis

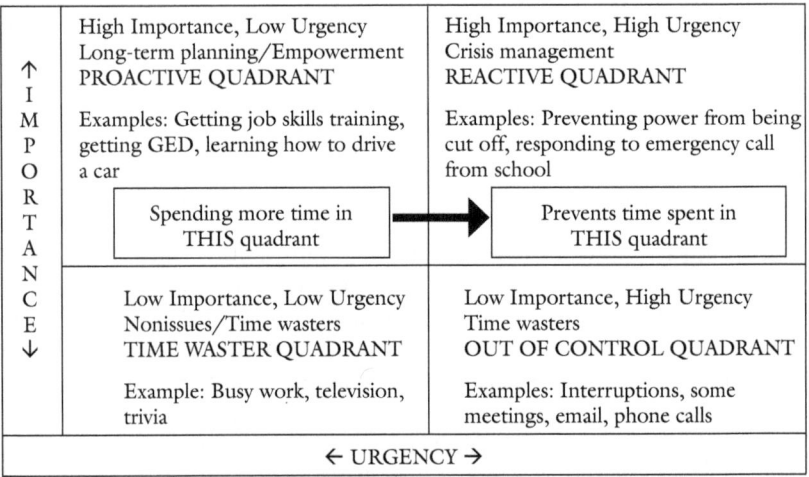

	High Importance, Low Urgency Long-term planning/Empowerment PROACTIVE QUADRANT Examples: Getting job skills training, getting GED, learning how to drive a car Spending more time in THIS quadrant	High Importance, High Urgency Crisis management REACTIVE QUADRANT Examples: Preventing power from being cut off, responding to emergency call from school Prevents time spent in THIS quadrant
↑ I M P O R T A N C E ↓	Low Importance, Low Urgency Nonissues/Time wasters TIME WASTER QUADRANT Example: Busy work, television, trivia	Low Importance, High Urgency Time wasters OUT OF CONTROL QUADRANT Examples: Interruptions, some meetings, email, phone calls
	← URGENCY →	

for what they have, what they do, and what they are capable of doing. We see Nancy and Alan encouraging the Stewarts to stretch their capabilities in ways that would empower them—to learn to drive a car, to change the way they handle their finances, to learn how to handle the family's emotional outbursts and the children's violent behaviors. Team members list strengths, acknowledge strengths, and use strengths to move the Stewarts and the team forward. They let the Stewarts do what they are capable of doing and enhance their capabilities with information and instruction. They use strengths of team members as they pool their talents and resources in ways that make the team feel supported and capable. They set goals with the family rather than for the family, and they help the family reach those goals by orally taking them through the steps necessary to do so. They listen to the family (and one another) and—rather than be put off by ways in which the family behaves differently than others do—take the effort to find out how the family's behaviors are logical responses to their environmental (and historical) situation. They focus on the future—on when and how things will be better—and thus transcend the past, which is laden with problems and deficits. They help when it will be helpful (empowering) to help, and they hold back help when it will be more helpful (empowering) not to help. Sometimes they help, but not with the type of help that is requested. In other words, the team is skilled and artful about giving and not giving help. By the end of the book, we've seen positive outcomes resulting from that kind of positive communication: Mrs. Stewart's crafts, Kevin's behaviors, and home improvements, among others.

In short, the team uses communication that empowers and enables the family by recognizing them as people who are capable, worthwhile, and valued; by seeing similarities rather than differences; and by looking for achievable but hopeful goals and dreams for the entire family.

This discussion rings up one last comment about enabling communication (see Davis, 2005). Although you want to use positive communication to help your clients to dream and to reach higher than their limiting view of the world might otherwise allow, possibilities and goals (desired outcomes) should be attainable and realistic. Is the goal within their control? Is it realistic to ask them to move toward this goal without determining if another desired outcome should be accomplished first? Given the current situation, should another, more attainable, outcome be set first? As Nancy and Alan did, it's also helpful to analyze the desired outcomes in terms of the present situation. What does the family have now, and how does what they want differ from what they currently have? One important question to ask is "why don't they already have this?" If you don't analyze what has been getting in their way of achieving this desired outcome thus far, you will be unable to identify and overcome the obstacles they will face in overcoming it in the future. Clearly, if this was an easy desired outcome for them to reach, they would have already reached it. How are they seeing this situation now, and how will they need to see it in the future in order to attain their desired outcome? These final questions lead to tangible action steps required to reach the desired outcome. First ask: "What resources do the family need to achieve this desired outcome?" These may take the form of money, support, tutoring, respite, and so on. Turn this list into actions by asking: "What actions will the team need to take to overcome these obstacles? How will it be possible to achieve this desired outcome?" Then list these as action steps along with the questions: "What specifically will we do to achieve this desired outcome? What steps will we take? When will we take them?" (Knight, 1995; Laborde, 1994; O'Conner & Seymour, 1990).

3. Therapeutic Relationship: Dialogue

Team members create a therapeutic relationship with the Stewarts, as I've said, through dialogic communication—communication at a deep level of meaning. Dialogue uses unconditional positive regard (strengths again) to nonjudgmentally acknowledge the other person and seeks to connect emotionally with the other. The team illustrates dialogue in many different ways. First, they empathize. They don't gloss over the family's problems, but they say that "they're doing the best they can" and find strengths that the family exhibits in the midst of their problems. Second, they recognize the common human connection between them and the Stewarts. They relate to the family in the ways in which they are the same, and they make the effort to see areas of commonality. Finally, they frankly care about the family and show that in the way they talk to them, talk about them, and interact with them. Having a team of people "on their side" helps the team and helps the Stewarts to move forward.

4. Facilitation Skills

Nancy's role of team leader is quite a challenging one. Hers is a peer-led team (Davis, 2008), in which the team leader leads an interagency team that includes team members at comparable levels in each of their respective organizations. The peer team leader has no formal power over the other members. The team leader typically has the daunting task of leading and coordinating a diverse team whose membership is fluid and whose members may have differing agendas and objectives, be without formal sources of power, and be from agencies that may represent conflicting mandates concerning children and families (Davis, 2008). Leading these teams requires an artful skill in facilitating meetings in a way that sets boundaries yet balances flexibility and structure in the team. In past research (Davis, 2005; Davis, Dollard, & Vergon, 2009) we've found several leadership and team behaviors that support child and family teams: creating a shared vision and mission for the team; choosing and articulating the outcomes desired for the family and the team; celebrating successes; recognizing the interconnectedness of the team members; and exerting boundaries over the team by introducing an agenda, guidelines, and/or ground rules for a meeting, or reviewing the system-of-care principles for team members.

Shared Vision and Mission   The first basic ingredient that successful teams require is a shared vision, a shared understanding of the way things will be. This vision represents the big picture of what the team is set to do, and the big-picture elements lead to an essential recognition: the mission is bigger than any one of the members—you can't do it alone. A strong vision and mission can draw people together. When group members all see the same vision, they can become a powerful force for change. A team vision gives your team something to work toward, together. The team in this research worked toward a common vision of the Stewart family, including Kevin, being successful and safe and positively functioning, at home and at school. To become a team, the team had to recognize that they couldn't achieve this mission without working together.

Desired Outcomes   Successful teams also require the creation of desired outcomes. Your team needs to agree on the outcomes toward which you are working. These would be the specific goals needed to improve Kevin's and the Stewarts' functioning at home and at school. Examples of desired outcomes for this team included Mrs. Stewart receiving her driver's license, Kevin's behavior improving at home and school, and the Stewarts' acquisition of a new home. Next, your team needs to divide your outcome into smaller, more manageable action steps—taking driving lessons, opening a checking account, creating and following a behavioral plan.

Celebrate Successes   You need to make sure to celebrate your team's successes. You need to use your team victories to motivate your team, and in these celebrations team members should emphasize the contributions made by each team member.

Recognize Interconnectedness   Systems thinking requires looking at your group through a wide-angle lens and realizing that the whole is made up of parts that are interconnected and interrelated. Unlike the traditional way of thinking of organizations in which groups are fragmented into separate parts (roles, jobs, organizations), systems thinking recognizes the relationships and interchanges among the different parts. It is systems thinking that creates cross-functional system-of-care teams, but, given the independent nature of the different entities that make up these teams, keeping this systems orientation is a challenge. It's important for the team to remember that—so far as their team is concerned—each part of the team exists only in relationship to the other parts; each part is what it is because of its context to the other parts. In a team, communication is the vehicle for establishing relationships and moving the team forward. If team members had one consistent criticism of the team as I conducted my interviews, it was that, between meetings, they wanted to be given more information about what was happening within the team.

For good or bad, in a system, one small event can have totally unforeseeable system-wide consequences—that's why Alan's intervention served as such a strong turning point for the team (Parker, 1994; Senge, 1994; Watzlawick, Bavelas, & Jackson, 1967; Wheatley, 1999). Therefore, if you don't like the way things are going on a team, change something—anything! Systems theory suggests that a change in the systems will ripple throughout.

Exerting Boundaries   Team members who have never been involved in a system of care before should be assimilated or socialized into the different expectations of the systems orientation. This socialization can occur through an agenda, meeting guidelines or ground rules, or an explanation of the systems-of-care principles.

A sample agenda that could be used for most wraparound meetings includes the following (see Davis, 2005) items:

1. Ground Rules
2. Strengths
3. Family Support Plan
4. Needs
5. Goals/Desired Outcomes
6. Action Steps
7. Assignments
8. Review
9. Adjourn

Even at a glance, this agenda tells participants what they can expect to happen in the meeting, and it shows them that the meeting will focus on family strengths, needs, and goals. If this agenda is sent out to participants before the meeting, they will come mentally prepared to fulfill their team roles. Also, including reminders of assignments from previous meetings will help participants to fully prepare for the meeting.

Meeting guidelines or ground rules also help to frame the meeting by making sure participants know up front what is expected of them. Once you have set the ground rules at the beginning of the meeting, it is easy to refer back to them later if someone breaks them ("Remember, we're focusing on strengths today!"). Here are some sample ground rules (see Davis, 2005) that you could send out with the agenda ahead of time.

1. Focus on strengths
2. Goals/Plan is based on family/child needs/strengths
3. Everyone is expected to contribute
4. Please avoid side conversations
5. Please avoid talking over others
6. Here's how we will be making decisions

You can also set the meeting expectations by your decision on where to hold the meeting and whom to invite to the meeting. A meeting in a nonprivate area of a school will feel much different from a meeting held in a parent's living room. Similarly, a meeting held with all school personnel will be very different from one held with all family friends or supports. You have more influence over the team location and attendees than you might realize. When making choices about a child and family team meeting, consider what is most conducive to the team process and what will best help you to meet your objectives for this meeting.

Team meetings can be classified into two categories: those that appear to be more tightly structured and those that are less structured. There appear to be both pros and cons to meeting structure. More structured meetings do seem to better reflect the system-of-care principles but may, by their structure, inhibit some team voices and ideas. However, less structured meetings may also inhibit voices and may be less oriented toward a system-of-care approach. It is not simply having a structure but the nature of the structure that is important in orienting the team toward a systems orientation. A structure that both overtly and covertly sets up the meeting within the system-of-care principles is the most effective in ensuring adherence to those principles. This structure can be accomplished by implicitly stating guidelines and rules and also by modeling those rules verbally and nonverbally (see Davis, Dollard, & Vergon, 2009).

5. Acknowledging Voice

The concept of power in these meetings is one of the key tensions I mentioned in an earlier chapter. The concept of power is tied up with the concept of voice. Being able to be heard is a key component of equal power in these teams. While all teams with families and formal system partners will always struggle with power issues (not only between providers and family but also between one provider and another), the family can be more equal partners on the team by having "voice." The team gives the Stewarts voice by listening to them, seeking to understand and respect them, and negotiating help with them rather than by imposing certain types of help on them.

For team members, including family members, to feel empowered, they must understand that they are both allowed to and capable of carrying out the group's mission. In the child and family team meetings, empowerment of the family might consist of helping them to build the skills required to take care of themselves, and, in fact, this is one of the stated goals of the system-of-care process. Adequate communication of the team and meeting principles goes a long way to fully empower the team. Helping team members feel a part of, and committed to, the group will empower them in the short term and the long term (Ashcraft & Kedrowicz, 2002; Müllern & Nordin, 2012; Orpen, 1997). Team members can be involved in setting meeting guidelines and rules (Arnold, 1996).

In addition, all team members, especially parents and informal supports, must be empowered by being both verbally and nonverbally encouraged to actively add input into the meeting process (Davis, 2008). You can empower your team members by understanding and acknowledging their strengths, helping them to create possibilities, encouraging them, staying positive, helping them to see their dreams, not "buying into" their excuses, helping them to think of ways things will work instead of ways they won't work; helping them to focus on concrete actions; helping them to focus on present successes and strengths; reminding them that they have choices; helping them to see how their actions create their circumstances; helping them to reframe their thoughts and attitudes; helping them to structure their goals, and asking them to report on their goals. This team clearly does all of these things for the Stewarts.

Conclusion

This research examines the construction of hope in a community mental health system of care. Groopman (2004) defines hope as the elevating feeling we experience when we see a path to a better future. In this in-depth study of a children's mental health system-of-care team, I find that members of the mental health care team create hope for themselves and for the family they are helping by using communication in specific ways. They maintain a strengths orientation and are future and possibility fo-cused. They move the family (and team) from crisis mode to empower-ment/proactive mode. They acknowledge, encourage, and enhance the capabilities of the family to promote and support their strengths focus. They coalesce as a team and pool their talents and resources to be more than they can be individually. They practice artful helping and not help-ing in ways that empower the family. They help the family dream yet set realistic goals to move them toward their dreams. They treat the family as people who are capable, worthwhile, and valued. They engage in dialogic communication at a deep level of meaning and interhuman connection. Using a common vision, mission, desired outcomes, and celebration of successes, they set boundaries to balance flexibility and structure. They give the family voice in the team and thus equalize power with the family. They do this through moments of empathy toward the family and other team members, engagement of all team members in the process, creation of a human connection within the team, vulnerability to one another, creation of possibilities for themselves and for one another, social sup-port, and blended voices. As the team moves forward in time and in team cohesion, they also move forward together in hope and empowerment. Constructing hope leads the family and team toward healing and motivat-ing, transcends the family's problems, and helps to empower and enable the family.

References

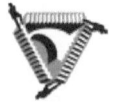

Anderson, R., Baxter, L. A., & Cissna, K. N. (2004). Texts and contexts of dialogue. In R. Anderson, L. A. Baxter, & K. N. Cissna (Eds.), *Dialogue: Theorizing difference in communication studies* (pp. 1–17). Thousand Oaks, CA: Sage.

Ardener, S. (1978). Introduction: The nature of women in society. In S. Ardener (Ed.), *Defining females* (pp. 9–48). New York: Wiley.

Arnold, V. (1996). Organizational development: Making teams work. *HR Focus, 73*(2), 12–14.

Ashcraft, K. L., & Kedrowicz, A. (2002). Self-direction or social support? Nonprofit empowerment and the tacit contract of organizational communication studies. *Communication Monographs, 69*, 88–110.

Averill, J. R., Catlin, G., & Chon, K. K. (1990). *Rules of hope.* New York: Springer-Verlag.

Barbee, A. P., & Cunningham, M. R. (1995). An experimental approach to social support communications: Interactive coping in close relationships. *Communication Yearbook, 18*, 381–413.

Barge, J. K. (2003). Hope, communication, and community building. *Southern Communication Journal, 69*, 63–81.

Barr, A., & Clark, D. (2010). Do the poor adapt to low income, minimal education, and ill health? *Journal of African Economies, 19*(3), 257–93; doi: 10.1093/jae/ejp024.

Barton, L. (1996). Sociology and disability: Some emerging issues. In L. Barton (Ed.), *Disability and society: Emerging issues and insights* (pp. 3–17). New York: Longman Publishing.

Baxter, L. A., & Montgomery, B. M. (1998). A guide to dialectical approaches to studying personal relationships. In B. M. Montgomery & L. A. Baxter (Eds.), *Dialectical approaches to studying personal relationships* (pp. 1–15). Mahwah, NJ: Lawrence Erlbaum.

Berg, I. K., & DeShazer, S. (1993). Making numbers talk: Language in therapy. In S. Friedman (Ed.), *The new language of change: Constructive collaboration in psychotherapy* (pp. 5–24). New York: Guilford Press.

Bickman, L., Smith, C. M., Lambert, E. W., & Andrade, A. R. (2003). Evaluation of a congressionally mandated wraparound demonstration. *Journal of Child and Family Studies, 12*, 135–56.

Bochner, A. P., & Eisenberg, E. M. (1987). Family process: Systems perspectives. In C. R. Berger & S. H. Chaffee (Eds.), *Handbook of communication science* (pp. 540–63). Beverly Hills, CA: Sage.

Bochner, A. P., Ellis, C., & Tillman-Healy, L. M. (1998). Mucking around looking for truth. In B. M. Montgomery & L. A. Baxter (Eds.), *Dialectical approaches to studying personal relationships* (pp. 41–62). Mahwah, NJ: Lawrence Erlbaum Associates.

Bogdan, R., & Taylor, S. J. (1989). Relationships with severely disabled people: The social construction of humanness. *Social Problems, 36*, 135–48.

Braithwaite, D. O., & Eckstein, N. J. (2003). How people with disabilities communicatively manage assistance: Helping as instrumental social support. *Journal of Applied Communication Research, 31*, 1–26.

Bronfenbrenner, U. (1979). Beyond the deficit model in child and family policy. *Teachers College Record, 81*, 95–104.

Brown, C. L., & Emery, J. (2010). The impact of disability on earnings and labour force participation in Canada: Evidence from the 2001 PALS and from Canadian Case Law. *Journal of Legal Economics, 16*(2), 19–59. Retrieved from EBSCOhost.

Bruner, J. (1990). *Acts of meaning*. Cambridge, MA: Harvard University Press.

Buber, M. (1965). *The knowledge of man: Selected essays* (M. Friedman & R. G. Smith, Trans.). London: Allen & Unwin.

Butterfield, R. M., & Lewis, M. A. (2002). Health-related social influence: A social ecological perspective on tactic use. *Journal of Social and Personal Relationships, 19*, 505–26.

Chen, S., Langner, C. A., & Mendoza-Denton, R. (2009). When dispositional and role power fit: Implications for self-expression and self-other congruence. *Journal of Personality & Social Psychology, 96*(3), 710–27; doi: 10.1037/a0014526.

Child Welfare and Juvenile Justice: Federal Agencies Could Play a Stronger Role in Helping States Reduce the Number of Children Placed Solely to Obtain Mental Health Services. (2003) *GAO Reports* (Vol. 1).

Cissna, K. N., & Anderson, R. (1990). The contributions of Carl R. Rogers to a philosophical praxis of dialogue. *Western Journal of Speech Communication, 54*, 125–47.

──────. (1998). Theorizing about dialogic moments: The Buber-Rogers position and postmodern themes. *Communication Theory, 8*, 63–104.

Cissna, K. N., Cox, D., & Bochner, A. P. (1989). Managing the dialectic between marital and parental relationships in the stepfamily. *Communication Monographs, 57*, 44–61.

Clark, D. A., & Qizilbash, M. (2008). Core poverty, vagueness and adaptation: A new methodology and some results for South Africa. *Journal of Development Studies, 44*(4), 519–44. Retrieved from EBSCOhost.

Clark, H. B., Lee, B., Prange, M. E., & McDonald, B. A. (1996). Children lost within the foster care system: Can wraparound service strategies improve placement outcomes? *Journal of Child and Family Studies, 5*, 39–54.

Clarke, R. T., Schaefer, M., Burchard, J. D., & Welkowitz, J. W. (1992). Wrapping community-based mental health services around children with a severe behavioral disorder: An evaluation of project wraparound. *Journal of Child and Family Studies, 1*, 241–61.

Cohen, S. G., & Bailey, D. E. (1987). What makes teams work: Group effectiveness research from the shop floor to the executive suite. *Journal of Management, 23*, 239–90.

Coles, R. (1989). *The call of stories: Teaching and the moral imagination*. Boston: Houghton Mifflin.

Conville, R. (1998). Telling stories: Dialectics of relational transition. In B. M. Montgomery & L. A. Baxter (Eds.), *Dialectical approaches to studying personal relationships* (pp. 17–40). Mahwah, NJ: Lawrence Erlbaum Associates.

Covey, S. R. (2004). *The 7 habits of highly successful people: Powerful lessons in personal change*. New York: Free Press.

Cutrona, C. E., & Suhr, J. A. (1992). Controllability of stressful events and satisfaction with spouse support behaviors. *Communication Research, 19*, 154–74.

Davis, C. S. (2005). Training curriculum: Strategic communication for effective wraparound facilitation. In C. Newman, C. Liberton, K. Kutash, & R. M. Friedman (Eds.), *The 17th annual research conference proceedings. A system of care for children's mental health: Expanding the research base* (pp. 173–77). Tampa: University of South Florida, The Louis de la Parte Florida Mental Health Institute, Research and Training Center for Children's Mental Health.

Davis, C. S. (2006) Sylvia's story: Narrative, storytelling, and power in a children's community mental health system of care. *Qualitative Inquiry, 12*(6), 1–24.

_____. (2008). Dueling narratives: How peer leaders use narrative to frame meaning in community mental health care teams. *Small Group Research: An International Journal of Theory, Investigation, and Application, 39*(6), 706–27.

Davis, C. S., & Dollard, N. (2004). THINK team observation: A mixed methods approach to assess service delivery in a community mental health system of care. In C. Newman, C. Liberton, K. Kutash, & R. M. Friedman (Eds.), *The 16th annual research conference proceedings. A system of care for children's mental health: Expanding the research base* (pp. 12–14). Tampa: University of South Florida, The Louis de la Parte Florida Mental Health Institute, Research and Training Center for Children's Mental Health.

Davis, C. S., Dollard, N., & Vergon, K. (2005). Negotiating practice: The use of communication to construct family-centered care in a community mental health system of care. In C. Newman, C. Liberton, K. Kutash, & R. M. Friedman (Eds.), *The 17th annual research conference proceedings. A system of care for children's mental health: Expanding the research base* (pp. 169–72). Tampa: University of South Florida, The Louis de la Parte Florida Mental Health Institute, Research and Training Center for Children's Mental Health.

_____. (2009). The role of communication in a child-parent-provider interaction in a children's mental health system of care. In T. J. Socha & G. H. Stamp (Eds.), *Parents, Children, and Communication II: Interfacing Outside the Home* (pp. 133–53). New York: Routledge.

Davis, C. S., Mayo, J., Piecora, B., & Wimberley, T. (2012). The social construction of hope through strengths-based health communication strategies: A children's mental health approach. In M. Pitts & T. Socha (Eds.), *Positive Communication in Health and Wellness* (pp. 63–81). New York: Peter Lang.

DeVito, J. A. (2001). *The Interpersonal Communication Book*. New York: Longman.

Duchnowski, A. J., Johnson, M. K., Hall, K. S., Kutash, K., & Friedman, R. M. (1993). The alternatives to residential treatment study: Initial findings. *Journal of Emotional and Behavioral Disorders, 1*, 17–26.

Dunst, C. J., & Trivette, C. M. (1996). Empowerment, effective helpgiving practices and family-centered care. *Pediatric Nursing, 22*, 334–37.

Dunst, C. J., Trivette, C. M., Davis, M., & Cornwell, J. C. (1994). Characteristics of effective help-giving practices. In C. J. Dunst, C. M. Trivette, & A. G. Deal (Eds.), *Supporting and strengthening families: Methods, strategies and practices* (pp. 171–85). Cambridge, MA: Brookline Books.

Dunst, C. J., Trivette, C. M., & Deal, A. G. (1994). Resource-based family-centered intervention practices. In C. J. Dunst, C. M. Trivette, & A. G. Deal (Eds.), *Supporting and strengthening families: Methods, strategies and practices* (pp. 140–51). Cambridge, MA: Brookline Books.

Dunst, C. J., Trivette, C. M., & Mott, D. W. (1994). Strengths-based family-centered intervention practices. In C. J. Dunst, C. M. Trivette, & A. G. Deal (Eds.), *Supporting and strengthening families: Methods, strategies, and practices* (pp. 115–31). Cambridge, MA: Brookline Books.

Durrant, M., & Kowalski, K. (1993). Enhancing views of competence. In S. Friedman (Ed.), *The new language of change: Constructive collaboration in psychotherapy* (pp. 107–37). New York: Guilford.

Eber, L., Nelson, C. M., & Miles, P. (1997). School-based wraparound for students with emotional and behavioral challenges. *Exceptional Children, 63*, 539–45.

Eber, L., Osuch, R., & Redditt, C. A. (1996). School-based applications of the wraparound process: Early results on service provision and student outcomes. *Journal of Child and Family Studies, 5*, 83–99.

Ekman, P., & Friesen, W. V. (1969). The repertoire of nonverbal behavior: Categories, origins, usage, and coding. *Semiotica, 1*, 49–98.

Ellis, C., & Bochner, A. P. (2000). Autoethnography, personal narrative, reflexivity: Researcher as subject. In N. K. Denzin & Y. S. Lincoln (Eds.), *The handbook of qualitative research* (pp. 733–68). Thousand Oaks, CA: Sage.

Faenza, M. M., & Steel, E. (1999). Mental health care coverage for children and families. In T. P. Gulotta, R. L. Hampton, G. R. Adams, B. A. Ryan, & R. P. Weissberg (Eds.), *Children's health care: Issues for the year 2000 and beyond* (pp. 117–35). Thousand Oaks, CA: Sage.

Fanger, M. T. (1993). After the shift: Time-effective treatment in the possibility frame. In S. Friedman (Ed.), *The new language of change* (pp. 85–106). New York: Guilford Press.

Farmer, P. (2003). *Pathologies of power: Health, human rights, and the new war on the poor.* Berkeley and Los Angeles: University of California Press.

Foucault, M. (1965). *Madness and civilization: A history of insanity in the age of reason.* New York: Random House.

————. (1995). *Discipline and punish: The birth of the prison* (A. Sheridan, Trans.). New York: Random House.

Frank, A. W. (1995). *The wounded storyteller.* Chicago: University of Chicago Press.

Friedman, R. M. (1994). Restructuring of systems to emphasize prevention and family support. *Journal of Clinical Child Psychology, 23* (Suppl.), 40–47.

Gergen, K. J. (1985). The social constructionist movement in modern psychology. *American Psychologist, 40*, 266–75.

————. (1999). *An invitation to social construction.* Thousand Oaks, CA: Sage Publications.

Gillis, J. (1996). *A world of their own making: Myth, ritual, and the quest for family values.* New York: Basic Books.

Groopman, J. (2004). *The anatomy of hope: How people prevail in the face of illness.* New York: Random House.

Guzzo, R. A., & Dickson, M. W. (1996). Teams in organizations: Recent research on performance and effectiveness. *Annual Review of Psychology, 47*, 307–38.

Haley, J. (1963). *Strategies of psychotherapy.* New York: Grune & Stratton.

Halfon, N., & Newacheck, P. W. (1999). Prevalence and impact of parent-reported disabling mental health conditions among U.S. children. *Journal of the American Academy of Child and Adolescent Psychiatry, 38*, 600–08.

Hammer, K., Mogensen, O., & Hall, E. O. C. (2009). The meaning of hope in nursing research: A meta-synthesis. *Scandinavian Journal of Caring Sciences, 23*(3), 549–57.

Hawes, L. C. (1994). Revisiting reflexivity. *Western Journal of Communication, 58*, 5–10.

Henderson, S. (2003). *A bitterness that transcends worlds: Exploring the social reality of suffering in illness.* Unpublished doctoral dissertation, University of California, Davis.

Henry, J. (1965). *Pathways to madness.* New York: Random House.

Hertz, R. (1997). Introduction: Reflexivity and voice. In R. Hertz (Ed.), *Reflexivity and voice* (pp. vii–xviii). Thousand Oaks, CA: Sage.

Hodges, S., Ferreira, K., Israel, N. (2012). "If we're going to change things, it has to be systematic": Systems change in children's mental health. *American Journal of Community Psychology, 49*(3/4), 526–37; doi: 10.1007/s10464-012-9491-1.

Hodges, S., Friedman, R. M., & Hernandez, M. (2008). Integrating the components into an effective system of care: A framework for putting the pieces together. In B. A. Stroul & G. M. Blau (Eds.), *The system of care handbook: Transforming mental health services for children, youth, and families* (pp. 71–94). Baltimore: Brookes Publishing.

Hoffman, L. (1981). *Foundations of family therapy.* New York: Basic Books.

Horwitz, A. V., & Scheid, T. L. (1999). Approaches to mental health and illness: Conflicting definitions and emphases. In A. V. Horwitz & T. L. Scheid (Eds.), *A handbook for the study of mental health* (pp. 1–11). New York: Cambridge University Press.

Jacobson, N. (2003). Defining recovery: An interactionist analysis of mental health policy development, Wisconsin 1996–1999. *Qualitative Health Research, 13*, 378–93.

Jarrett, R. L. (1992). A family case study: An examination of the underclass debate. In J. Gilgun, K. Daly, & G. Handel (Eds.), *Qualitative methods in family research* (pp. 172–97). Newbury Park, CT: Sage.

Jencks, C., Smith, M., Acland, H., Bane, M. J., Cohen, D., Gintis, H., Heyns, B., & Michelson, S. (2003). Inequality. In D. Conley (Ed.), *Wealth and poverty in America: A reader* (pp. 69–75). Malden, MA: Blackwell.

Johnson, S., & Long, L. M. (2002). Being a part and being apart. In L. R. Frey (Ed.), *New directions in group communication* (pp. 25–41). Thousand Oaks, CA: Sage.

Kaye, H. (2010). The impact of the 2007–2009 recession on workers with disabilities. *Monthly Labor Review, 133*(10), 19–30. Retrieved from EBSCOhost.

Kayser, T. A. (1994). *Building team power: How to unleash the collaborative genius of work teams.* Carlsbad, CA: Irwin Publishing.

Kearney, P. M., & Griffin, T. (2001). Between joy and sorrow: Being a parent of a child with developmental disability. *Journal of Advanced Nursing, 34*(5), 582–92.

Kelly, B. D. (2006). The power gap: Freedom, power, and mental illness. *Social Science & Medicine, 63*(8), 2118–128; doi: 10.1016/j.socscimed.2006.05.015.

King, G., Cathers, T., Brown, E., Specht, J. A., Willoughby, C., Polgar, J. M., MacKinnon, E., Smith, L. K., & Havens, L. (2003). Turning points and protective processes in the lives of people with chronic disabilities. *Qualitative Health Research, 13*, 184–206.

Knight, S. (1995). *NLP at work: The difference that makes a difference in business.* Sonoma, CA: Nicholas Brealey Publishing.

Kraus, M. W., Chen, S., Keltner, D. (2011). The power to be me : Power elevates self-concept consistency and authenticity. *Journal of Experimental Social Psychology, 47*(5), 974–80 ; doi : 10.1016/j.jesp.2011.03.017.

Laborde, G. Z. (1994). *Influencing with integrity : Management skills for communication and negotiation.* Mountain View, CA: Syntony Publishing.

Laveman, L. (2000). The Harmonium Project: A Macrosystemic approach to empowering adolescents. *Journal of Mental Health Counseling, 22*, 17–31.

Lezak, A., & MacBeth, G. (2002). *Overcoming barriers to serving our children in the community: Making the Olmstead decision work for children with mental health needs and their families.* Washington, D.C.: Center for Mental Health Services, Substance Abuse and Mental Health Services Administration, U.S. Department of Health and Human Services.

Liegghio, M., Nelson, G., & Evans, S. (2010). Partnering with children diagnosed with mental health issues: Contributions of a sociology of childhood perspective to Participatory Action Research. *American Journal of Community Psychology, 46*(1), 84–99; doi: 10.1007/s10464-010-9323-z.

Lincoln, Y. S., & Guba, E. G. (1985). *Naturalistic inquiry.* Newbury Park, CA: Sage.

Lipchik, E. (1993). "Both/And" solutions. In S. Friedman (Ed.), *The new language of change* (pp. 25–49). New York: Guilford Press.

Lourie, I. S. (2008). Foreword: The fantastic voyage. In B. A. Stroul & G. M. Blau (Eds.). *The system of care handbook: Transforming mental health services for children, youth, and families* (pp. xxix–xxx). Baltimore: Brookes Publishing.

Lourie, I. S., Katz-Leavy, J., & Stroul, B. A. (1996). Individualized services in a system of care. In B. A. Stroul (Ed.), *Children's mental health: Creating systems of care in a changing society* (pp. 429–52). Baltimore: Brookes Publishing.

Marks, D. (1999). *Disability: Controversial debates and psychosocial perspectives.* London: Routledge.

Martinez, A. G., Piff, P. K., Mendoza-Denton, R., & Hishaw, S. P. (2011). The power of a label: Mental illness diagnoses, ascribed humanity, and social rejection. *Journal of social and clinical psychology, 30*(1), 1–23; doi: 10.1521/jscp.2011.30.1.1.

Marvasti, A. B. (2002). Constructing the service-worthy homeless through narrative editing. *Journal of Contemporary Ethnography, 31*, 615–51.

Mayer, S. (2003). What money can't buy: Family income and children's life choices. In D. Conley (Ed.), *Wealth and poverty in America: A reader* (pp. 76–82). Malden, MA: Blackwell.

Miller, B., Blau, G., Christopher, O., & Jordan, P. (2012). Sustaining and expanding systems of care to provide mental health services for children, youth and families across America. *American Journal of Community Psychology, 49*(3/4), 566–79; doi:10.1007/ s10464-012-9517-7.

Minuchin, S. (1993). *Family healing: Strategies for hope and understanding.* New York: Free Press.

Mortola, P., & Carlson, J. (2003). "Collecting an anecdote": The role of narrative in school consultation. *The Family Journal: Counseling and Therapy for Couples and Families, 11*, 7–12.

Mullern, T., & Nordin, A. (2012). Revisiting empowerment: A study of improvement work in health care teams. *Quality Management in Health Care, 21*(2), 81–92; doi: 10.1097/ QMH.0b013e31824d18ee.

Myaard, M. J., Crawford, C., Jackson, M., & Alessi, G. (2000). Applying behavior analysis within the wraparound process: A multiple baseline study. *Journal of Emotional and Behavioral Disorders, 8*, 216.

Nelson, H. I. (2001). *Damaged identities, narrative repair.* Ithaca, NY: Cornell University Press.

O'Conner, J., & Seymour, J. (1990). *Introducing NLP: Neuro-linguistic programming. Psychological skills for understanding and influencing people.* San Francisco: Aquarian Press.

Oliver, M. (1990). *The politics of disablement: A sociological approach.* New York: St. Martin's Press.

Orbe, M. P. (1998). *Constructing co-cultural theory: An explication of culture, power, and communication.* Thousand Oaks, CA: Sage.

Orpen, C. (1997). The interactive effects of communication quality and job involvement on managerial job satisfaction and work motivation. *The Journal of Psychology, 131*, 519–22.

Owen, S. (2001). The practical, methodological, and ethical dilemmas of conducting focus groups with vulnerable clients. *Journal of Advanced Nursing, 36*, 652–58.

Parker, G. M. (1994). *Cross-functional teams: Working with allies, enemies, and other strangers.* San Francisco: Jossey-Bass.

Parkes, J. H., & Freshwater, D. S. (2012). The journey from despair to hope: An exploration of the phenomenon of psychological distress in women residing in British secure mental health services. *Journal of Psychiatric & Mental Health Nursing, 19*(7), 618–28; doi:10.1111/j.1365-2850.2012.01909.x.

Patterson, J. M. (2002). Understanding family resilience. *Journal of Clinical Psychology, 58*, 233–46.

Patton, M. Q. (2002). *Qualitative research and evaluation methods.* Thousand Oaks, CA: Sage.

Payne, H. (2009). Disabled children living away from home in the care system: Coordinating medical and health services. In C. Burns & C. Burns (Eds.), *Disabled children living away from home in the foster care and residential settings* (pp. 28–35). London: MacKeith Press.

Peterson, C. (1999). Psychological approaches to mental illness. In A. V. Horwitz & T. L. Scheid (Eds.), *A handbook for the study of mental health* (pp. 104–20). New York: Cambridge University Press.

Pettegrew, L. S., & Logan, R. (1987). The health care context. In C. R. Berger & S. H. Chaffee (Eds.), *Handbook of communication science* (pp. 675–710). Newbury Park, CA: Sage.

Polkinghorne, D. E. (1988). *Narrative knowing and the human sciences.* Albany: State University of New York Press.

Rawlins, W. (1983). Negotiating close friendship: The dialectic of conjunctive freedoms. *Human Communication Research, 9,* 255–66.

Ray, E. B. (1993). When the links become chains: Considering dysfunctions of supportive communication in the workplace. *Communication Monographs, 60,* 106–11.

Reed-Danahay, D. (2001). Autobiography, intimacy, and ethnography. In P. Atkinson (Ed.), *Handbook of ethnography* (pp. 407–25). Thousand Oaks, CA: Sage.

Richardson, G. E. (2002). The metatheory of resilience and resiliency. *Journal of Clinical Psychology, 58,* 307–21.

Richardson, L. (2000). Writing: A method of inquiry. In N. K. Denzin & Y. S. Lincoln (Eds.), *Handbook of qualitative research* (pp. 923–48). Thousand Oaks, CA: Sage.

Riley, S. E., Stromberg, A. J., & Clark, J. J. (2009). Relationship between caregiver hopefulness and satisfaction with their children's mental health services. *Community Mental Health Journal, 45*(4), 307–15; doi: 10.1007/s10597-009-9188-5.

Rosenfeld, L. B., Richman, J. M., & Bowen, G. L. (1998). Supportive communication and school outcomes for academically "at-risk" and other low-income middle school students. *Communication Education, 47,* 309–24.

Rotto, K., McIntyre, J. S., & Serkin, C. (2008). Strengths-based, individualized services in systems of care. In B. A. Stroul & G. M. Blau (Eds.), *The system of care handbook: Transforming mental health services for children, youth, and families* (pp. 401–35). Baltimore: Brookes Publishing.

Saleebey, D. (1996). The strengths perspective in social work practice: Extensions and cautions. *Social Work, 41,* 296–305.

Sari, H., & Altiparmak, S. (2012). Emotional burden of mothers of children with developmental disability. *Healthmed, 6*(1), 9–15.

Scheid, T. L., & Horwitz, A. V. (1999). Mental health systems and policy. In A. V. Horwitz & T. L. Scheid (Eds.), *A handbook for the study of mental health* (pp. 377–91). New York: Cambridge University Press.

Seligman, M., & Darling, R. B. (1997). *Ordinary families, special children: A systems approach to childhood disability.* New York: Guilford Press.

Sen, A. (1992). *Inequality re-examined.* Oxford: Oxford University Press.

Senge, P. M. (1994). *The fifth discipline: The art and practice of the learning organization.* New York: Doubleday.

Sherbourne, C. D., & Stewart, A. L. (1991). The MOS Social Support Survey. *Social Science and Medicine, 32,* 705–14.

Skiba, R. J., & Nichols, S. D. (2000). What works in wraparound programming. In M. P. Kluger & G. Alexander (Eds.), *What works in child welfare* (pp. 23–32). Washington, D.C.: Child Welfare League of America.

Skjorshammer, M. (2002). Understanding conflicts between health professionals: A narrative approach. *Qualitative Health Research, 12,* 915–31.

Snyder, C. R. (2000). The past and possible futures of hope. *Journal of Social and Clinical Psychology, 19,* 11–28.

_____. (2002). Hope theory: Rainbows in the mind. *Psychological Inquiry, 13*(4), 249.

Snyder, C. R., & McCullough, M. E. (2000). A positive psychology field of dreams: "If you build it, they will come." *Journal of Social and Clinical Psychology, 19,* 151–60.

Soundy, A., Smith, B., Butler, M., Lowe, C. M., Helen, D., & Winward, C. H. (2010). A qualitative study in neurological physiotherapy and hope: Beyond physical improvement. *Physiotherapy Theory & Practice, 26*(2), 79–88; doi: 10.3109/09593980802634466.

Stake, R. E. (1995). *The art of case study research.* Thousand Oaks, CA: Sage.

Stroul, B. A., & Blau, G. M. (2008). Introduction. In B. A. Stroul & G. M. Blau (Eds.). *The system of care handbook: Transforming mental health services for children, youth, and families* (pp. xxxvii–xxxix). Baltimore: Brookes Publishing.

Stroul, B. A., Blau, G. M., & Sondheimer, D. L. (2008). Systems of care: A strategy to transform children's mental health care. In B. A. Stroul & G. M. Blau (Eds.), *The system of care handbook: Transforming mental health services for children, youth, and families* (pp. 3–23). Baltimore: Brookes Publishing

Stroul, B. A., & Friedman, R. M. (1994). *A system of care for children and youth with severe emotional disturbances.* Washington, D.C.: Georgetown University Child Development Center, CASSP Technical Assistance Center.

Stylianos, S., & Kehyayan, V. (2012). Advocacy: Critical components in a comprehensive mental health system. *American Journal of Orthopsychiatry, 82*(1), 115–20; doi: 10.1111/j.1939.

Sykes, R. E. (1990). Imagining what we might study if we really studied small groups from a speech perspective. *Communication Studies, 41*, 200–11.

Szasz, T. (1970). *The manufacture of madness.* New York: Harper & Row.

—————. (1987). *Insanity: The idea and its consequences.* New York: John Wiley.

Tedlock, B. (2000). Ethnography and ethnographic representation. In N. K. Denzin & Y. S. Lincoln (Eds.), *The handbook of qualitative research* (pp. 733–68). Thousand Oaks, CA: Sage.

van Gestel-Timmermans, H., van den Bogaard, J., Brouwers, E., Herth, K., & van Nieuwenhuizen, C. (2010). Hope as a determinant of mental health recovery: A psychometric evaluation of the Herth Hope Index-Dutch version. *Scandinavian Journal of Caring Sciences, 24* (supplement 1), 67–74; doi: 10.1111/j.1471-6712.2009.00758.x.

VanDenBerg, J., Bruns, E., & Burchard, J. (2003, Fall). History of the wraparound process. *Focal Point: A National Bulletin on Family Support and Children's Mental Health, 17*, 4–7.

Walker, J. S., & Bruns, E. (2003, Fall). Quality and fidelity in wraparound. *Focal Point: A National Bulletin on Family Support and Children's Mental Health, 17*, 3.

Wall, C. J., & Gannon-Leary, P. (1999). A sentence made by men: Muted group theory revisited. *The European Journal of Women's Studies, 6*, 21–29.

Wampold, B. E., Ahn, H., & Coleman, H. L. K. (2001). Medical model as metaphor: Old habits die hard. *Journal of Counseling Psychology, 48*, 268–73.

Watts, E. K. (2001). "Voice" and "voicelessness" in rhetorical studies. *Quarterly Journal of Speech, 87*, 179–96.

Watzlawick, P., Bavelas, J. B., & Jackson, D. D. (1967). *Pragmatics of human communication.* New York: Norton.

Weber, M. (2003). The protestant work ethic and the spirit of capitalism. In D. Conley (Ed.), *Wealth and poverty in America: A reader* (pp. 29–42). Malden, MA: Blackwell.

Wheatley, M. J. (1999). *Leadership and the new science.* San Francisco: Berrett-Koehler.

Yoe, J. T., Santarcangelo, S., Atkins, M., & Burchard, J. D. (1996). Wraparound care in Vermont: Program development, implementation, and evaluation of a statewide system of individualized services. *Journal of Child and Family Studies, 5*, 23–37.

Yu, D. S. F., Lee, D. T. F., & Woo, J. (2004). Psychometric testing of the Chinese version of the Medical Outcomes Study Social Support Survey (MOS-SSS-C). *Research in Nursing and Health, 27*, 135–43.

Zola, I. K. (2004). *Missing pieces: A chronicle of living with a disability.* Philadelphia: Temple University Press.

Index

acknowledgment, 17, 86, 98, 167, 217, 221–22, 223, 227, 228
action steps, 93, 128, 223, 225, 226
agenda, 226
Asperger's autism, 110
at risk, 177

behavioral plan, 110, 128
biological approach to mental illness, 15
Bogdan and Taylor, 14
borrowed strengths, 105
boundaries, 103, 176, 189, 199, 201, 202–03, 212, 217, 224, 225, 228

case study, 20
child and family
    dreams or possibilities, 51, 54–56, 63, 105–06, 181–82, 185, 211, 213, 223, 227, 228
    interests, 105, 219
    positive behaviors, 84, 105, 128, 219
    positive traits, 105, 219
    resilience, 104, 105–07, 172, 219
Child and Family Branch of the Center for Mental Health Services (CMHS) in the Federal Substance Abuse and Mental Health Services Administration (SAMHSA), 215
child and family teams, 13–15
child-centered and family-focused care, 16
control, 14, 29–30, 49, 78, 106, 107, 108, 122, 150, 199, 202, 204
coping, 14
core poor, 26
crisis, 14, 16, 58, 59, 60, 62, 65, 155, 210, 221, 222, 228
crystallization, 20
cultural competence, 175, 185

culture, 15, 17, 18, 60, 104, 160–61, 165–66, 174–76, 182, 201, 216, 218

deficits, 15, 16, 17, 47, 104, 106, 107, 199, 218, 219, 220, 222
deficit-strengths tension, 30, 128, 199, 200, 202–03, 204, 211, 220
desired outcomes, 223, 224–25, 226, 228
despair, 14, 45, 55, 56, 199
deviance, 26, 27, 173–74
dialectical tensions, 198–99
dialogue, 201, 203–04, 211, 223
disabling, 199, 202, 221
disempower, 14, 16, 20, 107, 108, 123, 134, 169, 177, 199, 221
disenfranchisement, 45
dreams, 51, 54–56, 63, 105–06, 181–82, 185, 211, 213, 223, 227, 228

empathy, 167, 173, 174, 177, 199, 200, 203, 228
empowerment, 16, 20, 54, 58, 59, 78, 107, 108, 121, 123, 134, 135, 145, 155, 156, 177, 178, 181, 191, 192, 199, 202, 208, 217, 221, 222, 223, 227, 228
enabling, 106, 108, 219, 223, 228
environmental intervention/resources/ strengths, 106, 218–20, 222
ethics (research), 19, 21, 134, 212
evocative narrative, 21

family
    as full participants, 57, 62, 125, 170, 216
    competencies/strengths, 55, 56, 105–07, 111, 218–21
    empowerment, 121
    involvement, 105, 216
    resources, 17

support plan, 24, 226
system, 53, 54, 59, 99, 164, 166, 169, 216
team, 17, 19, 20, 54, 59, 66, 77, 177, 191–92, 199, 218, 220, 224
voice, 155, 217
family-centered, 78, 146, 210
focus group, 20, 65–92, 138–49, 188–213
Foucault, 16, 111
future tense, 104, 204

goals, 219, 220, 221, 222, 223, 224, 226

hegemony, 107
helping versus not helping, 98, 107, 108, 109, 120, 123, 228
hope, 14, 54, 59, 76, 77, 78, 79, 93, 97, 98, 104, 105, 106, 107, 109–10, 112, 140, 145–46, 159, 171, 172–73, 176, 179, 182, 189, 192, 195, 199–200, 201–02, 204, 211, 213, 219–21, 228
false hope, 172–73, 199–200
hope theory, 105
hopelessness, 14, 44, 45, 47, 54, 112, 199–200
humanness, 14, 89, 201

illness viewpoint of mental illness, 15
individualized care, 16, 78, 109, 192, 210, 216
informal supports, 13, 210, 216, 227
information broker, 114
interhuman connection, 200, 203, 211, 228

labeling, 16, 111
life domains, 99

marginalization, 14, 45
medical model, 14–17, 57, 111
medical terminology, 111
meeting
   facilitation, 217, 224
   guidelines or ground rules, 224–27
   structure, 227
mission, 224, 227–28
muting/muted group, 14, 167

narrative, 20–21
naturalistic setting, 19
nonverbal communication, 72, 82, 179, 227

objectivity, 19
outcomes, 98, 120, 199, 200, 210, 217, 222–25, 228

pathology, 98, 174
peer team leader, 224
positive
   communication, 78, 113, 115, 133, 145, 196, 220, 223
   feelings, attitudes, and values, 105, 208, 219, 220
   focused interventions, 84, 106, 107, 128, 133, 218, 219, 220
   outcomes, 98, 105, 106, 126, 127, 128, 199, 200, 211, 217, 218, 219, 220, 222
   traits, 105, 219
possibilities, 16, 54, 104–07, 199–200, 203, 211, 218, 219, 220, 227
poverty, 24–27, 45, 168
   and parenting, 26–27
   core poor, 26
   culture/environment of poverty, 25, 45
   moral dimension, 25
power, 13, 14, 16, 47, 54, 62, 107, 116, 122, 125, 134, 155, 156, 170, 178, 199, 201, 224, 227, 228
problems, 15, 17, 28, 30–31, 33, 45, 47, 51, 52, 55, 57, 59–60, 62, 70, 82, 105, 106, 109, 114, 116, 126, 128, 130, 148, 168, 169, 174, 183, 185, 192, 195, 202, 203, 211, 218–21
progress, 180
psychological view of mental illness, 15

reflexivity, 19
research rigor, 20
resiliency, 104–07, 172, 219
Richardson, Laurel, 20

safety, 31–32, 59, 86–87, 90, 97, 99, 102, 104, 110, 124, 128, 150, 178, 202
safety plan, 91, 96, 101, 103, 155
school psychologist, 136, 159, 161, 170
SED (Severe Emotional Disturbances), 12–13
shared vision, 224
sick role, 15
social constructionism, 14, 18, 27
   and parenting, 27
   and poverty, 27
   of humanness, 14

social support, 19, 108, 200, 228
Soft Systems Methodological Approach
    (SSM), 210
solution talk, 106
stigma, 15, 168
strengths
    behavioral strengths, 105, 219
    borrowed strengths, 105, 106, 107, 219,
        220
    environmental strengths, 105, 106, 219,
        220
    hidden strengths, 105, 107, 117, 219,
        220
    historical strengths, 105, 219
    interest strengths, 105, 219
    past strengths, 105, 106, 107, 219, 220
    positive feelings, attitudes, and values,
        105, 107, 219, 220
    possibility, dream, or future strengths,
        105, 106, 107, 191, 219, 220
    resilience, 105, 107, 219
    resource strengths, 105, 107, 219, 220
    talent strengths, 105, 107, 219
    trait strengths, 105, 219
strengths approach/orientation/
    perspective/language, 16, 17, 28, 29,
    31, 45, 47, 55–56, 57, 61, 77, 78, 79,
    98, 104, 105, 128, 134, 145, 192, 199,
    200, 203, 205, 217, 218, 219, 222, 223,
    226, 227

strengths-deficit tension, 30, 104, 199,
    202, 203, 204, 211
system of care, 12, 13, 14, 15, 16, 17, 18,
    20, 98, 147, 210, 215, 216, 217
    team leader, 19, 57, 100, 224
    teams, 18, 210, 211, 218, 225, 227
systems theory, 32, 34, 164, 216, 225
systems-based approach, 45, 70, 93,
    100–01, 169, 210, 225

team approach, 13, 14, 15, 16, 17, 18,
    120–21, 123, 124, 142, 147, 177, 209
team-based organizing, 18
therapeutic environment, 103, 217
therapeutic relationship, 217, 218, 223
traditional medical model, 15
trust, 172, 176
turning point, 80, 93, 121, 122, 135, 206,
    225

unconditional positive regard, 173, 223

voice, 17, 19, 21, 34, 54, 62, 86, 98, 116,
    122, 155, 156, 167, 199, 200, 201, 204,
    210, 217, 227, 228
vulnerability, 20, 108, 122, 177, 199, 200,
    203, 204, 211, 228

About the Author

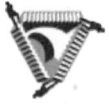

Christine S. Davis, Ph.D., is an Associate Professor in the Communication Studies Department at the University of North Carolina at Charlotte. Before coming to UNCC, she was a researcher at the Louis de la Parte Florida Mental Health Institute at the University of South Florida, where she was involved in numerous projects that studied the communication processes involved in children's mental health services. She also developed and conducted dozens of training sessions on wraparound team meeting facilitation. At the University of North Carolina at Charlotte, Dr. Davis is involved in several community research and service projects studying communication among patients with disabilities and terminal prognoses, and their families and providers. Her research interests are in the intersection of family, health, and disability. Dr. Davis publishes regularly on topics such as children's mental health, end-of-life communication, family disability, spirituality and health care, and narrative ethnography and autoethnography. Her B.A. degree in Communication is from Virginia Polytechnic Institute and State University (Virginia Tech); her M.A. degree in Communication Studies is from the University of North Carolina at Greensboro; and her Ph.D. in Communication Studies is from the University of South Florida.